Legal and Ethical Issues in Health Occupations

Second Edition

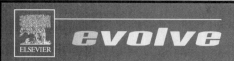

Legal and Ethical Issues in Health Occupations

Second Edition

Tonia Dandry Aiken, RN, BSN, JD
Attorney at Law
New Orleans, Louisiana

President and Co-founder—Nurse Attorney Institute, LLC
Louisiana State University Health Sciences Center School of Nursing—Adjunct Faculty
  Legal Nurse Consultant Program
A Past President of The American Association of Nurse Attorneys and the Foundation

SAUNDERS

ELSEVIER

SAUNDERS
ELSEVIER

11830 Westline Industrial Drive
St. Louis, Missouri 63146

LEGAL AND ETHICAL ISSUES IN HEALTH OCCUPATIONS,
SECOND EDITION

ISBN: 978-1-4160-2262-6

Notice

Neither the Publisher nor the Author assume any responsibility for any loss or injury and/or damage to persons or property arising out of or related to any use of the material contained in this book. It is the responsibility of the treating practitioner, relying on independent expertise and knowledge of the patient, to determine the best treatment and method of application for the patient.

The Publisher

Library of Congress Control Number 2007940528

Publishing Director: Andrew Allen
Acquisitions Editor: Jennifer Allen
Developmental Editor: Kelly Brinkman
Publishing Services Manager: Melissa Lastarria
Senior Project Manager: Joy Moore
Senior Designer: Andrea Lutes

ISBN: 978-1-4160-2262-6

Printed in the United States of America.
Last digit is the print number: 9 8 7 6 5 4 3

To my loving husband, Jim, and our wonderful children, Brett, Alexes, and Candace, who gave me support and encouragement.

To my parents, Shirley and Anthony Dandry, who taught me to reach for the sky and go after my dreams.

To Tina, Larry, Kyle, and Matthew Mayes; Julie and Courtney Bounds; Kathy Moisewicz; Jean Farquharson; Sally, Jack, Lynn and Larry Aiken; and Rita, Ragus, Andrea and Ali Legendre for always being there.

To Diane Warlick, RN, JD, my good friend and business partner.

And to Theresa Nicholson, my friend and assistant.

Contributor

Ruth Ann Ehrlich, RT (R)
Adjunct Faculty
Portland Community College
Portland, Oregon

Preface

The purpose of the second edition of *Legal and Ethical Issues in Health Professions* is to provide allied health professionals with a textbook and reference that focuses on the legal and ethical issues faced by them in daily practice in a user-friendly format. Features such as Case Examples and "What If" Boxes focusing on legal and ethical dilemmas aid the healthcare professional in developing critical thinking skills to resolve issues they may encounter in their practices.

The approach of this book is to provide three units that build on one another. The sections progress from basic legal principles and doctrines to specific chapters on each of the allied health professions. For example, Unit I, *Legal Issues,* discusses topics such as the law, intentional and quasi-intentional torts, professional liability insurance, informed consent issues, and documentation.

Unit II, *Ethical Issues,* is an introduction to ethical issues in health occupations and discusses those issues affecting educators and students.

Unit III, *Common Areas of Liability and Litigation,* features a revised chapter, "Legal and Ethical Considerations in Medical Imaging." This chapter explains the principles of ethics that apply to medical imaging personnel. Unit III also covers administrative and medical records, laboratory, medical equipment, patient care, and conflict management.

The following features are included in the chapters to be used as learning tools:
• Key Chapter Concepts
• Objectives
• Introduction
• Case Examples
• Case Discussions
• Pertinent Points
• Study Questions
• References
• Resources

New features to this edition include:
- Information on HIPAA and its ethical and legal implications
- "What If" Boxes—added throughout text to present students with real-life ethical dilemmas; each box is followed by three critical-thinking questions
- Updated Case Studies—more applicable for a 21st-century audience

This book is designed as a basic legal textbook and is appropriate for graduate or advanced levels of allied health professional students, practicing allied health professionals, nurses, physicians, attorneys, administrators, and other healthcare professionals.

In addition to the book, this edition also has an accompanying Evolve® Website. This resource features many useful teaching tools for instructors such as a 250-question test bank, sample legal documents, additional case studies, PowerPoint slides, an Instructor's Manual, and a TEACH lesson plan manual that will incorporate the Evolve® Resources alongside the book so that instructors will have a ready-to-use cohesive lesson plan for each chapter.

Tonia Dandry Aiken, RN, BSN, JD

Acknowledgment

I want to thank the talented and knowledgeable contributors, friends, and colleagues who gave their valuable time and expertise to help in the creation of this needed text and resource book. Also, thanks to Jena Henning with the California State Department of Health Services.

Also, I would like to thank Brett and Alexes, who were part of my research and support team.

Also, a warm thanks to Jennifer Presley, Kelly Brinkman, Lynda Huenefeld, Loren Wilson, and Richard Hund for their guidance in producing our book.

■ Additional Acknowledgments

I would especially like to thank the talented and knowledgeable contributors from the first edition of this book who helped build the foundation for this edition:

James B. Aiken, MD, MHA, FACEP
Associate Professor of Emergency Medicine of Public Health—LSU Health Science Center, Medical Director of Emergency Preparedness at LSU University Hospital in New Orleans, New Orleans, Louisiana

Mary Powers Antoine, RN, JD
Partner Nossman, Gunthner, Knox & Elliott, LLP
Sacramento, California

Linda Auton, RN, JD
President, Auton Law Offices, PC, Rockland, Massachusetts

Nancy Cline, RDH, MPH
Blanco, Texas

Barbara Edwards, RN, MTS
Arlington, Virginia

Jean Farquharson, RN, JD
Attorney at Law, Bradenton, Florida

Ardele Float, RN, JD
Attorney at Law, Georgia

Kathleen M. Gialanella, RN, JD, LLM
Attorney at Kathleen M. Gialanella, PC, Westfield, New Jersey

Paula Dimeo Grant, RN, BSN, MA, JD
Attorney at Law, Washington, DC

Patricia Iyer, RN, MSN, LNCC
President, Med League Support Services, Inc, Flemington,
New Jersey

Britta E. LaFont, RDH, BA, Med
New Orleans, Louisiana

M. Lee Leppanen, RN, JD
Attorney at Law, Concord, New Hampshire

Joann Pietro, RN, JD
Warhenberger & Pietro, LLP, Springfield, New Jersey

Gloria C. Ramsey, RN, JD
Associate Professor, Uniformed Services University of the Health
Sciences, Bethesda, Maryland

Jan Simoneaux, RN, MN
Director of Nursing for Nursing Professional Development—
Ochsner Medical Center, New Orleans, Louisiana

Diane Trace Warlick, RN, JD
Co-founder—Nurse Attorney Institute, LLC, Louisiana State
University Health Sciences Center School of Nursing—Adjunct
Faculty - Legal Nurse Consultant Program, A Past President of
The American Association of Nurse Attorneys and the Foundation,
Dallas, Texas

Contents

Legal Issues

The Law

Key Chapter Concepts

- Administrative Law
- Admissions of Fact
- Appellate Court
- Civil Code
- Civil Law
- Common Law
- Criminal Law
- Defendant
- Executive Branch
- Felony
- Good Samaritan Laws
- Interrogatories
- Judicial Branch
- Jurisdiction
- Law
- Legislative Branch
- Malpractice
- Misdemeanor
- Negligence
- Plaintiff
- Request for Production of Documents
- Res Ipsa Loquitur
- Respondeat Superior
- Sources of Law
- Sovereign Immunity
- Stare Decisis
- Statute of Limitations
- Supreme Court
- Tort

Objectives

At the conclusion of the chapter, the reader will be able to:

1. Define the sources and types of laws.
2. Describe the differences among the executive, judiciary, and legislative branches.
3. Discuss the different levels of the judicial system.
4. Discuss the four elements of negligence.
5. Define common legal concepts and terms.

■ Introduction

Every job, profession, and career has a distinct vocabulary. Once you are familiar with the vocabulary, the ideas, concepts, and structure of the job become understandable. This chapter reviews the major legal concepts and terms that aid in the understanding of the concepts in the text and how those concepts affect a healthcare provider.

■ What Is the Law?

Law is the foundation of statutes, rules, and regulations that govern people, relationships, behaviors, and interactions with the state, society, and federal government. It provides order in resolving conflicts among individuals, corporations, states, and other entities. The goal of the law is to resolve disputes without violence and to protect individual citizens' health, safety, and welfare.

The law, although based on solid, long-held tenets, customs, and beliefs, is constantly evolving and growing to meet the changes, challenges, and constant shifts of our society. For example, the past century has seen minorities empowered by laws changed to meet the ever-evolving social, political, and personal values of society.

■ Sources of Law

The foundation of the law of the land is the Constitution. It grants certain powers to the federal government. If the power is not expressly granted to the federal government, then it is reserved to the state government.

The constitutional basis for federal involvement in health care is found under the provision for the general welfare and regulation of interstate commerce. The states have the power to regulate health care through their police power to protect the health, safety, and welfare of their citizens. This includes the regulation of nurses, pharmacists, physicians, chiropractors, physical therapists, and other licensed healthcare providers.

The Constitution and the Bill of Rights guarantee certain fundamental freedoms to individuals. They affect the healthcare system by providing the fundamental rights to **privacy, equal protection, freedom of speech,** and **religion.**

The three branches of government provide the other sources of law (Box 1-1). They are the **legislative, executive,** and **judicial branches.** The first branch, the **legislature,** develops **statutory law.** These laws are codified and impact all citizens of the state. The Medicare and Medicaid amendments to the Social Security Act of 1965 have dramatically affected health care, particularly in the services available in hospitals, communities, and at home; in hospital admissions and discharges; and in the level of care provided.

The second branch of government is the **executive branch.** The President or state governor proposes laws, vetoes laws proposed by the legislature, and enforces the laws. The executive branch also proposes and establishes agencies.

Agencies, under the direction of the executive branch, enact rules and regulations that become **administrative law.** Once the legislature creates a statute, it empowers the agency to implement and establish rules and regulations to meet the intent of the statute. These rules and regulations codify the interactions between the citizens and the agencies, provide for certain police power to the agencies to enforce the regulations, and govern the agencies themselves. For example, **Occupational Safety and Health Administration (OSHA)** rules apply to most workplaces, including healthcare facilities. Another agency that regulates healthcare

Box 1-1 | Four Sources of Law

1. Constitution and Bill of Rights
2. Common law or case law, from the judicial branch
3. Statutory law, from the legislatures
4. Administrative law, from the executive branch

workplaces is the Department of Public Health (DPH), which surveys nursing homes, hospitals, and other healthcare facilities to establish regulations and to enforce compliance with those regulations. The nurse practice acts of the various states create administrative agencies, such as the state boards of nursing, which have the authority to make and enforce rules and regulations concerning nursing practice. Likewise, the boards of medical examiners enforce rules and regulations that affect medical practice.

The third branch is the **judicial system,** which develops and interprets the statutory law. It is also the source of common law, which is the law that develops from the decisions made by courts. Previous decisions are considered **precedent** and binding on all lower courts. In Latin this is called **stare decisis,** which means to "stand by things decided" or "adhere to decided cases."

Common law originated from England with the Pilgrims and original settlers of the land. Since that time, each state's courts have made decisions regarding civil and criminal cases.

■ Checks and Balances

Our government has developed into three separate branches. The **executive branch** is the President of the United States or governor of an individual state. This branch also includes agencies that execute the laws passed by the legislature. The **legislative branch** is the **House of Representatives** and **Senate** of the United States and any similar legislature of a state. The **judicial branch** is the court system. This system includes the federal courts and state courts.

Each branch serves as a **check and balance** for the other branches of government (Box 1-2). The legislature proposes and passes statutes and can override the veto of the President or

Box 1-2 | Checks and Balances

- *Executive branch:* President or governor, can veto legislation and enforces the laws
- *Legislative branch:* proposes and passes legislation; can override the President or governor
- *Judicial branch:* interprets legislation; can overrule laws and actions of the executive branch

governor. The court can declare laws that the legislature develops unconstitutional, and it interprets the laws. The governor or President can propose or veto legislation, appoint or nominate individuals to the court, and enforce the laws. This interaction provides the checks and balances for each branch.

The legislature proposes and passes laws that govern the individual states, the citizens, and residents of the country and enables certain agencies to develop rules and regulations. These **rules and regulations** developed by agencies such as the Environmental Protection Agency (EPA), the Board of Registration in Nursing, the Board of Registration of Physicians, and OSHA apply to many employees in the healthcare field.

The court system interprets those laws passed by the legislature as they are applied in individual cases. The court also interprets regulations and their application to individual cases, but not until all remedies provided by the regulations are exhausted. For example, the Board of Registration of Pharmacists and the employer of Brett, a pharmacist, accuse Brett of drug diversion. After a hearing, the board suspends Brett's license as a pharmacist. Brett may appeal the case to the court. However, if there was not a hearing, Brett cannot appeal to the court, as he has not exhausted his remedies.

■ Types of Law

Common Law

The law can be classified in many ways. One way is to look at its origins. Common law is derived from English common laws or written civil code (Box 1-3). These legal principles were developed when the king pronounced rules on the basis of his "divine right." Case decisions were accumulated and based on reason and justice. All the states, except for Louisiana, have adopted the common law system. Because each state adopted different statutes and judicial interpretations, variations of the law exist among the states.

Only Louisiana, originally colonized by France, adopted a civil code based on the Napoleonic Code. The code is law created by the

Box 1-3 | Common Law Versus Civil Code

- *Common law:* developed on a case-by-case basis from England when the king decided on the basis of his "divine right"
- *Civil code:* developed from Roman law codified by the legislature

legislature rather than the judiciary. It is a comprehensive written set of rules and regulations rather than case-by-case analysis and interpretation of legal issues. It is based on Roman, Spanish, and French civil laws, not on English common law.

■ Civil Law Versus Criminal Law

Another way to classify law is whether there is a **civil wrong** (often called a **tort**) that causes harm to a person or a person's property or a **criminal wrong** that violates criminal statutes (Box 1-4).

Lawsuits against healthcare providers can be **criminal** or **civil.** The distinction is the remedy or penalty, often called a **sanction.**

Civil law encompasses various areas of law, including but not limited to contract issues, intentional torts, and negligence, malpractice, labor, and privacy issues. Most cases against healthcare workers are for **negligence** or **malpractice.** The allegations in the suit are often that the healthcare provider failed to provide care that met the standard of care and that harm resulted to the patient. The **remedies** (Box 1-5) in civil law are almost exclusively monetary. The court cannot impose servitude or

Box 1-4 | Civil Law Versus Criminal Law

- *Civil law:* case brought by an individual or entity against another individual or entity for harm based in tort, contract, labor, or privacy issues
- *Criminal law:* case brought by the state or federal government for violation of written criminal code or statute

Box 1-5 | Remedies

- *Civil remedies:* usually monetary award
- *Criminal remedies:*
  1. Misdemeanors: lesser fines and jail time of less than one year
  2. Felonies: major fines and jail time of more than one year, or the death penalty (in some states)
- *Administrative remedies:*
  1. Monetary fines
  2. Required education
  3. Loss of license to practice

make the plaintiff "whole" again when the plaintiff has suffered such things as loss of a limb, pain, or emotional problems. The monetary award is an attempt to make the person "whole" again. On rare occasions, the court may order a person to stop doing something until a full hearing is held on an issue, to prevent harm from occurring that money cannot remedy.

Criminal law is concerned with violations against society based on the criminal statutes or code. The remedies for the state or federal government are monetary fines, imprisonment, and death. **Misdemeanors** are lesser crimes punishable by (usually modest) fines established by the state and/or imprisonment of less than one year. **Felonies** are more serious crimes punishable by much larger fines and/or imprisonment for more than one year or, in some states, death. In many states, a felony conviction may be the grounds for revoking a license to practice in a healthcare field. A healthcare provider may be prosecuted criminally for practicing without a license, falsifying information in obtaining a license, failing to provide life support for terminally ill patients, or abusing a patient.

-- ■ ■ ■ **What If?**

You are assigned to a different unit to work with the nursing staff. The nurse you are assigned to is the best friend of your sister. She is often missing from the unit and you cannot find her to report on your patients.

You report to her that the blood pressure is high for Mrs. Nicholson and that she says her head hurts. You report the information to the nurse, who then disappears. A half hour later, you walk into the room and Mrs. Nicholson is drooling and has paralysis on the left side of her body. The nurse comes up to you and begs you not to tell the nurse manager that you reported an elevated blood pressure and headache because she is on probation.

1. What are the ethical implications?
2. Are the four elements of negligence found in this scenario?
3. Are there issues that can affect the licenses of the healthcare providers?

An agency may have both civil and criminal aspects to its rules and regulations. The remedies available encompass more than either civil or criminal law. For example, the various boards of registration can probate, suspend, or revoke an individual's license to practice. The boards can also impose educational requirements; require fines, periodic supervisor evaluations, and drug and alcohol screens (if abuse or diversion is an issue); place restrictions on areas of practice; and require a recovery program or Alcoholics

Anonymous/Narcotics Anonymous meetings, as well as evaluations by a psychologist, psychiatrist, and/or addictionist. Certain agencies may have other remedies that are specific to the agency and may vary greatly from agency to agency. For example, the DPH can suspend an institution's ability to receive Medicare or Medicaid funding, which are the major sources of funding for hospitals, rehabilitation centers, and nursing homes, as well as impose major fines. Medicare and Medicaid fraud can also lead to incarceration.

■ The Court System

Each state has several levels of courts. The local courts usually handle crimes and civil cases that do not exceed a certain minor monetary sum established by the legislature.

The next level of court is a court with general jurisdiction, which is the major trial court with broad powers. It is in this court that medical malpractice, elder abuse, negligence, major crimes, and other civil wrongs are tried.

Sometimes there may be specific courts that handle exclusively family or probate (generally dealing with wills and administering estates) cases, juvenile cases, housing issues, or land issues. They are limited in their jurisdiction to only specific types of cases.

To try a specific case, the court must have **jurisdiction** (Box 1-6) over the case. Jurisdiction can be **in personam** or **in rem**. **In personam** jurisdiction means the court has jurisdiction over the person. For example, the major trial courts' jurisdiction is based on county lines or other such divisions. If the action giving rise to the case occurred in the county or parish, the trial court in that county or parish has jurisdiction over the case and the people involved. The plaintiff may have the option of bringing the case in his or her own county or parish, depending on the rules of procedure for that state. In certain instances, the plaintiff may have to file a case where the defendant lives, such as in cases involving collection of money owed.

In rem jurisdiction means the court has jurisdiction over the property or thing itself rather than over the people involved.

Box 1-6 | Jurisdiction

- *In personam:* the court has jurisdiction or control over the person.
- *In rem:* the court has jurisdiction or control over the thing or property.

The court determines the right to the specific property, which is binding usually against the whole world, not just the parties involved.

Once a trial is completed or a case is final in the court of general jurisdiction, or in one of the specific courts, a case may be appealed to a higher court, usually called an **appeals court** or an **appellate court**. There are both state and federal appellate courts. An **appeal** may only raise an issue of law. The facts, as found by the jury or the judge, cannot be appealed. If the appeals court decides a case and no further appeal is taken, the appellate decision is binding on all lower courts in the state.

From the state appeals court, an appeal may be taken to the top court of the state, usually called the **State Supreme Court.** Again, only issues of law can be appealed. The State Supreme Court does not act on most cases, and the parties have no recourse for further review unless a **writ of certiorari** is filed with the U.S. Supreme Court and the Court chooses to hear the case. The ruling by the U.S. Supreme Court is binding on all state courts.

Some cases may be filed and tried in **federal district court.** There are 94 judicial districts organized into 12 regional circuits. Each circuit has a U.S. Court of Appeals (Box 1-7).

The Justices choose the cases that the U.S. Supreme Court hears. The party appealing the lower federal court's decision or a state supreme court's decision with a federal question files a petition called a writ of certiorari. The U.S. Supreme Court chooses very few cases to hear. Those that are chosen must involve a question of substantial importance. For example, the case *Roe v. Wade* posed the question as to whether the constitutional rights of women and of developing embryos and fetuses require that abortion be legal for some portion of the pregnancy. Once the U.S. Supreme Court decides a case, it is binding on all state and federal courts.

Box 1-7 | The U.S. Federal Courts

- U.S. Supreme Court
- U.S. Court of Appeals (Appellate Court)
  - 12 Regional Circuit Courts of Appeals
  - 1 U.S. Court of Appeals for the Federal Circuit
- U.S. District Courts (Trial Courts)
  - 94 Judicial districts
  - U.S. Bankruptcy Court

■ Definitions

The name of a case indicates who is suing whom. The person or entity bringing the suit is called the **plaintiff.** For example, the patient who brings a complaint against the hospital, healthcare provider, or facility is the plaintiff. The person or entity who is sued and defending against the allegations is the **defendant.** The plaintiff is listed first in the **caption** and the defendant is listed after the *versus* (v.), such as *Alexes and Kyle Andrea v. Alexandra Hospital.*

■ Latin Terms

Certain terms in law come from Latin. The term **tort** comes from Latin, meaning "to twist, be twisted, or to wrest aside." **Tort** is a private or civil wrong or injury, and not a breach of contract, for which the court provides a remedy for damages. There must always be a violation of some duty owed to the plaintiff, and generally such duty must arise by operation of law and not by mere agreement of the parties.

Respondeat superior means "let the master answer." If a nursing assistant is sued for actions that harm a patient, her employer can also be sued. The employer can be sued on the basis that the employer had control, or should have had control, over the actions of the nursing assistant and that the nursing assistant was working in the course and scope of her employment.

Res ipsa loquitur means "the thing speaks for itself." For example, a person has surgery to correct a hernia, but when he awakes, his arm is paralyzed. Because he had no control over his actions during the surgery and a paralyzed arm is not an expected outcome or even a possible adverse reaction, then the law presumes that the paralysis had to be caused by the negligence of the surgical technician, operating room nurse, surgeon, and/or anesthesiologist. This presumption means that the plaintiff does not have to prove that negligence occurred in order to recover from the defendant.

Stare decisis means "to stand by things decided." This prevents multiple suits on the same facts with the same parties. It allows courts to refer to previously decided similar cases and to apply the same rules and principles. The courts can follow prior decisions or those of courts of higher jurisdiction.

■ **Other Terms**

Negligence is a tort. It is the cornerstone of a **malpractice** case. Negligence does not require a specific plan to harm someone. There are four elements in a negligence action: duty, breach of duty, proximate harm or causal connection, and harm/damages (Box 1-8), which will be discussed in depth later.

Case Discussion

Facts: A 75-year-old patient at a licensed healthcare provider care center suffered from diabetes, dementia, coronary artery disease, immobile decubitus ulcers (bedsores), and was unable to walk, talk, or feed herself.
 	
    Her physician prescribed a daily whirlpool bath as a medical treatment for the decubitus ulcers. The facility did not have a whirlpool so she was given a regular daily bath. A certified nursing assistant prepared a bath for the patient and placed her in hot water that was 138 degrees and that subsequently caused severe burns from which she died three days later.
 	
    A wrongful death action was brought. Parties settled before trial for $1.5 million.
 	
    Source: *Strine v. Commonwealth of Pennsylvania, et al.*, 894 A.2d 733 (Pa. 2006).
1. Are all of the elements of negligence in the above case?
2. Discuss the breaches of the standard of care.
3. How could the patient's death have been prevented? How could a safer environment have been provided?

   Malpractice requires proof of a breach of a standard of care, and the breach must cause damage or harm. *Malpractice* is a term used to describe the negligence of professionals, including healthcare providers. You will hear it most often in reference to nursing, medicine, and law.

Box 1-8 | Elements of Negligence

1. Duty
2. Breach of the duty
3. Proximate cause (causal connection)
4. Harm/damages

A **statute of limitations** requires that a case be brought within a specific time limit. The requirement varies from state to state. In some states a suit must be filed within one to three years from the act or discovery of negligence or malpractice. Check your specific state statute and Federal Tort Claims Act for cases filed in federal courts. Different causes of action have different statutes of limitations. The expiration of the statute of limitations is a defense to a lawsuit.

▪ ▪ ▪ **What If?**

You are asked to lie about the time your coworker came in to work. She told you she was late because she had to tube feed her terminally ill mother. You know for a fact that she was at the local department store because you overheard a phone call to her friend.
1. What is the ethical thing to do?
2. What are the other implications if you lie for her?
3. What are the facility's policies and your professional ethics statement on falsification of documents?

Insurance seems easily definable. It is a contract between the insured and the insurer that protects the insured from a specified loss. For example, a healthcare provider purchases a **professional liability policy**, also known as **malpractice insurance,** in case she negligently injures a patient and is sued. The plaintiff receives only money for the injury and the insurance company pays the defense costs to attorneys and any monetary award for the plaintiff. In consideration for paying the policy premiums, the insurance company will make these payments on behalf of the insured. Many insurance companies have both professional liability insurance and **disciplinary defense insurance** (to pay for costs of defending against a complaint made to the healthcare provider's board.)

Good Samaritan laws protect those who provide health care for an emergency or disaster without reimbursement. If a nursing assistant stops at an automobile accident and helps the victims, without seeking payment, and is not grossly negligent in rendering care, then the law covers the nursing assistant.

Sovereign immunity is a defense that protects a federal or state employee when acting within the scope of employment. This defense is eroding.

Discovery
1. **Interrogatories** are written questions that must be answered in writing under oath. They are part of the discovery process to prepare for mediation, settlement, and trial.

2. **Requests for Production of Documents** are a discovery tool whereby requests are submitted to the opposing party to produce specified documents or items that are pertinent to the issues of the case.

3. **Admissions of Fact** are a discovery technique that asks the opposing party (in writing) to admit or deny any material fact or the authenticity of documents to be introduced into evidence at trial.

This chapter is merely a brief introduction to the terms and concepts found in this text. For further information regarding the terms, see the corresponding chapters.

■ ■ ■ Pertinent Points

1. The goal of the law is to settle disputes without violence.
2. The three branches of state and federal governments are judicial, legislative, and executive.
3. The four sources of law are the Constitution, common law, the legislature, and administrative law.
4. The plaintiff is the person or entity suing. The defendant is the person or entity sued and defending against allegations.
5. When a plaintiff sues a defendant in a malpractice suit, it involves civil law.
6. Medical malpractice claims are based on tort theory. A tort is a civil wrong that causes harm or injury.
7. Civil law remedies provide primarily monetary damages.
8. Criminal law remedies include fines, incarceration, and possibly a death sentence.
9. Administrative law governs the rules and regulations of the different agencies and enforces them.
10. Administrative law remedies include fines, education, and restrictions on areas of practice and restrictions on the healthcare provider's license.
11. The legal doctrine of respondeat superior is used to hold the employer responsible and liable for the negligent acts of its employees as long as the employee is working within the course and scope of employment.
12. The doctrine of res ipsa loquitur shifts the burden of proof from the plaintiffs to the defendants, who then must defend their position.
13. Good Samaritan laws protect those who provide health care in an emergency without payment.

■ ■ ■ Study Questions

1. Discuss the reasons and goals of the law.
2. Discuss how the law changes.
3. Discuss the sources of the law and their interactions.
4. Describe the differences between civil, criminal, and administrative law.
5. Discuss the differences among the executive, judiciary, and legislative branches.
6. Go to the law library or use the internet to obtain a copy of an actual case in your area of practice. (Use recommended websites.)
7. Describe the different levels of the judicial system.
8. Define the following terms: plaintiff, defendant, and jurisdiction. From the case you obtained, identify each.
9. What are the four elements of negligence? Underline each element you find in the case you obtained.
10. How do Good Samaritan laws protect a healthcare worker?
11. Discuss the elements of a case that fall under the doctrine of res ipsa loquitur.
12. Discuss a criminal case involving a healthcare provider.
13. Define five grounds for disciplinary actions in your area of practice.
14. Discuss the types of administrative law remedies that you have seen in your area of practice.
15. Obtain the contact information and services provided by your board of registration.

■ ■ ■ Resources

www.findlaw.com
www.lexisone.com
www.nurselaw.com
www.usa.gov
www.uscourts.gov

2

Intentional and Quasi-Intentional Torts

Key Chapter Concepts

- Assault
- Battery
- Consent
- Defamation
- False Imprisonment
- Intent
- Intentional Infliction of Emotional Distress
- Intentional Tort
- Invasion of Privacy
- Quasi-Intentional Tort
- Sexual Assault or Misconduct with Patients
- Trespass to Land

Objectives

At the conclusion of this chapter, the reader will be able to:

1. Define the nature of intentional and quasi-intentional torts and how they differ from negligence or strict liability.
2. Discuss the necessary intent needed to commit an intentional or quasi-intentional tort.
3. Discuss the elements of intentional and quasi-intentional torts.
4. Define the importance of consent.
5. Discuss defenses to intentional and quasi-intentional torts.
6. Discuss the legal and ethical implications of Health Insurance Portability and Accountability (HIPAA).

■ Introduction

In day-to-day practice, healthcare professionals confront situations in which they must perform invasive, sometimes painful, and often-humiliating procedures on their patients. Under different circumstances, these actions can give rise to legal actions against the healthcare professional. While most healthcare professionals think of negligence or malpractice actions, there is another area of law where potential liability rests. It is the area known as **intentional and quasi-intentional torts.**

■ Definition of a Tort

A **tort** is a civil wrong other than breach of contract. The word *tort* is derived from an Old Norman word meaning "wrong." **A tort is a harm against a person, whereas a crime is a harm against the state.** For example, someone steals your purse. You file a complaint with the police, and the police arrest John Jones for the crime of theft. When Jones goes to court, the case is titled *State v. John Jones.* The state brings the action because a crime is deemed a harm against the peace and tranquility of all persons in the state, not just the victim.

If a tort is committed, however, an individual brings the case against another individual. The state does not have an interest in seeing that you are paid money damages for any loss you sustained. In the above example, you can bring a civil action against John Jones for any loss you sustained in the theft of your purse. In such an action, you seek money damages for the loss.

Almost all torts can be crimes, but most crimes are not torts. If prison is the penalty, then the action is a crime. If money damages are the penalty, then the action is a tort.

There are four types of torts: **negligence, intentional torts, quasi-intentional torts,** and **strict liability.** The essence of negligence is a breach of established standards of care, whereas the essence of strict liability is the relationship to or ownership of the thing that caused harm. The essence of intentional and quasi-intentional torts is consent.

■ Intentional Torts

The major intentional torts are **assault, battery, false imprisonment, intentional infliction of emotional distress,** and in specific areas of nursing such as home care, **trespass to land.** Broadly defined, intentional torts require that there be an intentional interference with an individual's person, reputation, or property.

Intent

The degree of **intent** necessary to commit an intentional tort is broader than having a desire to bring about harm or injury to a person. If a person is or should be substantially certain that given circumstances will follow from his actions, then there exists the requisite intent. For example, if you walk behind a healthcare provider in the hospital just as he pulls a tray from the dinner cart and hits you, there is no intent to harm you, and no intentional tort is committed. But if a healthcare provider takes the tray and throws it across the room at a patient's bed so that it hits the patient, then he knew or should have known that the action of throwing a tray was likely to hit someone and cause injury. That knowledge is sufficient to form the intent necessary to commit an intentional tort of assault and battery in this case.

Intent may also be transferred. For example, you intend to shoot person A, but you miss and shoot person B instead. Even though you have no intent to harm person B, your intent to harm person A is transferred, and the law deems that you had the intent to harm person B. It is a rule of law that "intent follows the bullet." While transferred intent does not often occur in the medical setting, if a healthcare provider gives the wrong patient an injection, she can be liable for battery and negligence even though she has no intent to harm that patient or any conscious desire to administer the injection to the wrong patient.

To be liable for an intentional tort, a person must meet all elements of the tort. If any one element is missing, then no tort has been committed. Each of the specific torts mentioned above has specific elements that must be met.

Assault

An **assault** means placing someone in immediate fear or apprehension of a harmful or noxious touching without the patient's consent. To commit an assault, the person must be aware that you are about to touch him or her.

For example, a patient is in bed crying and becomes hysterical. The home health aide caring for the patient becomes increasingly anxious and upset as a result of the patient's behavior. The aide raises her hand over her head and threatens to strike the patient. (The aide does not have to tell the patient anything; raising the hand as if to strike is enough.) If the patient sees the aide raising her hand and cringes to protect herself, then the patient is put in imminent fear of a battery, and the aide commits an assault.

If, on the other hand, the patient is crying into her pillow and does not see the aide raise her hand to strike, then the patient is not put in fear of an imminent battery and no assault is committed.

Usually, however, an assault precedes a battery, and the two torts are often grouped together. Keep in mind, however, that they are two separate torts.

Battery

A **battery** is harmful or offensive touching of another without his or her consent or without a legally justifiable reason. Without the consent of the patient, or absent an emergency, any touching of a patient can be a battery.

A battery does not mean you must try to maliciously hurt or strike a person. Any touching, such as inserting an intravenous device, may be a battery if done without the consent of the person or without a legally justifiable reason. Also, hitting, spitting at, kicking, and slapping a patient can all be batteries. In addition, you do not need to touch the patient to commit a battery. If you touch something in close proximity to the person without his or her consent, then a battery is committed. For example, if a patient wants to leave the hospital against medical advice and as the healthcare provider you grab her purse or suitcase from her hand, you have committed a battery. Even though your intent may have been noble (i.e., protecting her health by keeping her in the hospital), you have committed a battery.

Case Discussion

Facts: A certified nursing assistant was involved in an altercation with an Alzheimer's patient who suffered injuries including hematomas near the eyebrows and a skin tear on her forearm along with bruises to the face and neck and around the eyes.

The trial court rendered a judgment against the medical center for $40,000 and against the nursing assistant for $25,000.

The Tennessee Court of Appeals at Nashville affirmed the trial court's decision against the nursing assistant and reversed the judgment against the medical center because the Government Tort Liability Act does not permit the plaintiff to sue the medical center for the nursing assistant's intentional tort. (The plaintiff's claim was based on the legal doctrines of negligent retention or vicarious liability.)

Note: A claim for negligent retention was based on the plaintiff's claim that the medical center had prior notice of the nursing assistant's propensity for violence on the basis of an earlier incident.

The Supreme Court of Tennessee held that the harm arising from the intentional acts of the nursing assistant was a foreseeable risk created by the negligent medical center. The Court held that each tortfeasor part was jointly and severally liable for the entire amount of damages awarded. The Court reversed in part and affirmed in part the Court of Appeals and remanded the case to the Circuit Court to determine the total amount of damages to be awarded to the plaintiff.

Source: Limbaugh v. Coffee Medical Center, 59 S.W. 73 (Tenn. 10/16/2001).

Consent

A **battery** is any offensive touching without permission or in the absence of an emergency situation. All patients admitted to a hospital are required to sign a general consent. This general consent is for medical care and treatment for other employees of the hospital to "touch" the patient, even in a therapeutic manner. Do not confuse this **general consent** with an **informed consent** to surgery or to other invasive procedures. While the failure to obtain an informed consent may give rise to an action in medical negligence, the consent necessary to avoid a battery is the permission to touch the person.

A medical **battery** can be committed in specific situations where there is consent to perform some procedure but you perform another. At the cornerstone of this theory is the decision of the brilliant jurist Justice Benjamin Cardozo, who wrote in 1914: "Every human being of adult years and sound mind has a right to determine what shall be done with his own body, and a surgeon who performs an operation without his patient's consent commits an assault for which he is liable in damages" [1].

While you may think that no person would perform a procedure other than the one authorized, several cases are instructive. In *Pizzaloto v. Wilson*, the patient gave consent for the surgeon to perform exploratory surgery to accomplish lysis of adhesions and fulguration of endometriosis [2]. During the abdominal surgery, the physician noted that the plaintiff's reproductive organs had sustained severe damage. He determined that she was in fact sterile and proceeded to perform a total hysterectomy and bilateral salpingo-oophorectomy.

When the plaintiff awoke from surgery, she was upset with what the physician had done. In ruling in her favor, the court ruled that the plaintiff was entitled to recover damages because there was no emergency present and the surgeon committed a battery. The court awarded her $10,000. See also *Guin v. Sison*, where the court awarded $1000 to a postmenopausal women who had her left fallopian tube and ovary removed without consent during the course of a colectomy [3].

Female patients are not the only ones who need be concerned. In a recent Pennsylvania case, plaintiff sought defendant's assistance for treatment of premature ejaculation [4]. After conservative treatment gave only temporary relief, the defendant suggested a surgery to clear out plaque from the plaintiff's penis. Upon awakening from surgery, the plaintiff was given a warranty card by the nurse for the penile implant the defendant had inserted during surgery. It was undisputed that no consent was given for the implant. While the trial court originally dismissed the claim because the plaintiff did not have an expert witness, the appeals court reversed and ordered the trial court to proceed with the case.

In each of the examples given, the physicians defended on the basis that they were protecting the patients from the need for a second surgery. Even if true, and even though the physicians performed both surgeries skillfully, the courts still held that the decision to undergo specific surgery is the plaintiff's, and absent an emergency, a physician cannot exceed the scope of the patient's consent. If the physician does so, he or she commits a battery.

Physicians are not the only ones who commit medical battery. Consider the facts of *Roberson v. Provident House*, where plaintiff, a quadriplegic, was admitted to defendant nursing home [5]. Plaintiff wore a condom catheter, but the nursing staff obtained an order to insert a Foley catheter as needed. The order was obtained because occasionally problems developed with the condom catheter and the patient leaked urine. The physician did not discuss the insertion of a Foley catheter with the plaintiff, and the plaintiff was unaware that the order was written.

On two separate occasions the Foley catheter was inserted over the objections of the plaintiff, despite his repeated requests to have the catheter removed. After the second insertion, when the plaintiff complained bitterly each shift, one nurse, who was tired of the plaintiff's complaints, jerked the catheter out, causing a discharge of blood and pus. The court found the nursing staff and their employer liable for battery. The plaintiff was awarded $25,000.

This case teaches several lessons. First and foremost, if your patient refuses to allow you to perform a procedure, **stop.** If the patient objects after the fact and you can remedy the situation, then do so. In no event should any healthcare provider proceed with any procedure without the unwavering consent of the patient. Next, never perform a procedure for the convenience of the staff. That is not a reason to violate the patient's right to refuse.

-■ ■ ■ **What If?**

A patient needs to receive a barium swallow but refuses to swallow the contrast medium. The hospital worker in charge of the patient takes the cup and forces the patient to drink it. You are an employee and you see what has happened.
1. Has an intentional or quasi-intentional tort been committed?
2. What are your legal and ethical responsibilities as an employee?
3. Does the patient have any rights?

Implied Consent

There are limited situations in which the courts imply consent on behalf of the plaintiff. In one of the oldest cases of implied consent, the plaintiff, an employee of defendant, spoke no English. He was standing in line with other employees to be vaccinated. He asked no questions. He watched others being vaccinated, and when it was his turn, he held up his arm to the physician who proceeded with the vaccination. When plaintiff filed suit against the company and others alleging battery, the court stated the plaintiff's action clearly indicated **implied consent or implied permission** to touch him. The court dismissed the battery claim [6]. It is highly unlikely that any similar situation would arise in medicine today, but there are circumstances when **consent will be implied.**

In modern medicine, consent is implied in **emergency situations.** The situation must be life threatening or pose a risk of significant physical injury to the patient if the procedures are not performed. Only those procedures absolutely necessary are authorized, and as soon as possible competent consent should be obtained. Only a physician can make the determination that a true emergency exists that necessitates proceeding without consent.

Ethical dilemmas can arise for healthcare professionals when treating individuals who, for **religious reasons,** do not allow certain procedures to be performed. If the physicians are aware of the patient's religious beliefs, then consent is not implied. If the physician is not aware, then the courts will most likely rule that consent is implied, as long as the physician had no way of knowing the religious prohibitions.

If the religious prohibitions are known, then consent is not implied, even in the case of a minor. In *Novak v. Cobb County Kennestone Hospital Authority,* the hospital obtained a court order to administer blood to a 16-year-old Jehovah's Witness [7]. The order was entered despite the protest of the boy and his mother. Even though the mother and child brought suit after the boy had recovered, the court dismissed all claims. Without the court order, however, the hospital and physicians could not have proceeded with the blood transfusions. Keep in mind that a court will only order procedures in the case of a minor. If a competent adult refuses life-saving treatment, the courts will not interfere, nor will they imply consent.

To prevent allegations of battery, always have your patient's written consent to perform a procedure. Only perform the procedure authorized, and do not exceed the scope of the consent. In emergency situations, have at least two physicians certify that an emergency exists, document the certification in the patient's record, and perform only those procedures that are necessary to save a person's life or to prevent significant injury or harm. As soon as possible, obtain competent consent for the performance of additional procedures.

All states have statutes that outline when consent is implied. Healthcare providers must be aware of what their individual state laws are and, as advocates of the patient's rights, do all in their power to see to it that the law is followed.

Sexual Assault or Misconduct with Patients

The American Medical Association's Council of Ethical and Judicial Affairs has banned sexual conduct with patients under the guise of treatment in Opinion 8.14A (www.ama-assn.org/ama/pub/category/8503.html). The American Psychiatric Association has ruled that under no circumstance is sexual activity between therapist and patient permissible. The reasons for these prohibitions are clearly illuminated in the classic case of sexual misconduct with a patient, *DiLeo v. Nugent* [8]. In *DiLeo,* plaintiff was a patient of the defendant psychiatrist for several months. In an effort to work through an impasse in therapy, the psychiatrist suggested she undergo therapy with the use of the date-rape drug ecstasy. She and her psychiatrist had an "all day experimental session" with the plaintiff using ecstasy and tryptamine to boost the effect of the ecstasy. While plaintiff was under the influence of the drug, defendant repeatedly had sexual contact with her. Defendant was found liable not only of negligence but also of willful misrepresentation. Plaintiff was awarded $500,000. (Although plaintiff did not sue under a theory of assault and battery, the facts of *DiLeo* clearly support those claims.)

Psychiatrists are not the only physicians who have been sued for sexual misconduct. In *Smith v. St. Paul Fire and Marine Insurance Co.,* plaintiffs sued a family practitioner for sexually assaulting three boys he was treating for conditions totally unrelated to their sexual organs [9]. In *St. Paul Fire and Marine Insurance Co. v. Asbury,* several women sued a gynecologist for fondling their clitoris during routine gynecological examinations [10]. And in *St. Paul Fire and Marine Insurance Co. v. Shernow,* a dentist was sued for giving a female patient excessive doses of nitrous oxide and then sexually assaulting her [11]. No matter what theory of liability, under no circumstances are medical practitioners, nurses, or allied health personnel to have sexual relations with their patients.

▪ ▪ ▪ **What If?**

A patient has approached you about dating him. You have been caring for this patient off and on for 4 years.
1. What should you do?
2. Is it okay to date him? Why or why not?

False Imprisonment

False imprisonment is the unlawful detention of a person. The person is deprived of his personal liberty of movement against his will and without any authority to detain. To be falsely imprisoned, a person must be confined within a specific area against his will; he must be confined by means of physical barriers and/or by physical force or threat of physical force, and he must be aware of the confinement.

Issues of false imprisonment generally arise in three circumstances: first, in the psychiatric setting with involuntary commitments; second, with the use of restraints, either physical or chemical; and third, in situations where a patient attempts to leave the hospital against medical advice.

In the psychiatric setting, the most important defense to a claim of false imprisonment is that all requirements in law of an involuntary admission are met. Requirements that must be met include the following:
1. The statutory provisions for the reason for involuntary commitment, such as danger to self or others, exist.
2. All statutory requirements for physician examination have been met in a timely manner.
3. All appropriate documentation exists in the chart to support the action of involuntary admission.
4. All the patient's rights have been followed.

5. All statutory time limits have been met but not exceeded for holding an individual against his will.

The following cases demonstrate the right and wrong ways to effect an involuntary admission.

In the case *Brand v. University Hospital*, the plaintiff was out of town when she became ill [12]. As she was driving to the local hospital, she experienced a seizure, blacked out behind the wheel, and was involved in an accident. She was transported from the scene of the accident to the local hospital. In the emergency department, the treating physician gave her the option of being admitted to neurological service for a workup or of being discharged to her home to follow up with her own neurologist. Plaintiff opted for the latter.

Because of her medical condition she called friends to drive her home. One of her co-workers, a former drug addict, assumed the patient's behavior was due to a drug problem, and she brought the patient to the behavioral treatment unit of University Hospital. The patient was so groggy she fell asleep and did not realize where she was.

The next morning when the plaintiff woke up and realized she was in a locked psychiatric ward, she asked to be transferred to a medical ward of the hospital. She requested that the physician call the other hospital and call her neurologist. Neither the physician nor hospital staff listened to the plaintiff for more than 36 hours. The trial court originally dismissed the plaintiff's claim, but the appeals court overturned that decision and plaintiff was allowed to proceed against the hospital staff and physician.

The statutory requirements for an involuntary admission were not met. There was no documentation that the patient was a danger to herself or others. There was insufficient physician examination. The staff of the behavioral unit had no right to detain the plaintiff without properly and timely obtaining appropriate release information.

In contrast, in *Mawhirt v. Ahmed*, plaintiff brought suit against the hospital, physicians, and nurses for false imprisonment secondary to an involuntary admission and the use of both physical and chemical restraints [13]. The difference between this case and *Brand* is that the physicians and staff had well documented the severe psychiatric state of the patient. The plaintiff was suffering from paranoid delusions that the CIA and Mafia were out to get him. Two physicians determined he was a danger to himself and others and proceeded with the appropriate procedures for the involuntary admission.

The nursing staff documented the psychotic, delusional behavior of the plaintiff as well as behavior by which the plaintiff could harm himself or threaten other patients. They followed the institution's guidelines for the administration of chemical restraints and the procedures set out for the use of physical restraints. As such, the court had no difficulty in dismissing plaintiff's claims.

Documentation of the behavior necessitating the use of restraints is critical. Under no circumstances are restraints to be used for the convenience of the staff to control an unruly patient. Your institution's policy must be clear as to:
1. The circumstances under which restraints may be used;
2. How they are to be used and for how long;
3. What type of monitoring the patient will require;
4. What documentation is adequate to justify the use of these restraints; and
5. How often the physician must reorder the use of physical restraint.

Inadequate proof of the patient's condition or need for an involuntary admission was an issue in *Davis v. St. Jude Medical Center* [14]. Plaintiff was a patient on a medical unit for the treatment of pancreatitis. Approximately three weeks after this admission, a staff physician involuntarily admitted him to the hospital's chemical dependency unit. Plaintiff repeatedly requested to be released. He even put his request in writing to the hospital's administration. He brought a habeas corpus hearing but was discharged before the hearing took place. He then brought an action for **false imprisonment.** In allowing the patient to proceed with his action, the court ruled that the hospital and physicians had failed to provide the court sufficient proof of the necessity of the patient's involuntary admission or necessity of treatment. It is important to make certain that all the requirements have been met, documented, and made part of the medical record.

Use of restraints is not limited to the psychiatric setting. In many hospitals and nursing homes, patients are restrained to prevent injury. **Even putting up side rails on a bed is a form of restraint.** The reasons that, for example, side rails are up should be documented in the record. If the patient refuses to allow the side rails to be put up, then have her sign a release from liability in the event of a fall. Even though it is probably not worth the paper it is written on in a court of law, a release gives the patient the opportunity to appreciate the gravity of her decision to refuse the side rails. **Use of any other type of restraint, such as sheets to hold patients in wheelchairs, posey belts, or any other form of**

physical restraint, should be used only as a last resort and must be used only as approved by hospital policy and the physician. In all situations when possible, obtain written consent for the use of any type of restraint.

Home Care Setting

In the home care setting, it is highly recommended that home care personnel do not place patients in restraints. Home care personnel are not available for a sufficient amount of time to evaluate the patient's response to the restraints, to evaluate the need for continued use of restraints, to determine whether the restraints are being used properly, or to determine how the patient is being monitored while in restraints. If the family puts the patient in restraints, notify the physician, obtain an order, and instruct the family of the proper care of a patient in restraints.

Against Medical Advice

Another situation that raises possible issues of false imprisonment involves patients wishing to leave the hospital against medical advice (AMA). While you may talk to a patient about the consequences of the decision to leave and you have an obligation to review with the patient all the possible complications that could arise should he leave AMA, you cannot prevent a competent patient from refusing treatment or leaving. This means you cannot physically bar the patient's exit. You cannot prevent the patient from getting his clothes or other personal belongings, and you cannot attempt to touch the patient in an effort to make him stay.

In a particularly egregious case, a 67-year-old man was physically prevented from leaving a nursing home for 51 days [15]. Shortly after his nephew admitted him to the nursing home, the man attempted to leave. Nursing home employees forcibly returned him. The man continued to demand his release and made several additional attempts to leave the home. He was finally placed in a restraint chair and denied use of the phone or even access to his own clothes. The court found that the actions of the staff were in complete and utter disregard of the man's rights and were willful, reckless, and malicious in detaining him. **Where the patient is competent, he cannot be detained against his will.**

If a situation exists where the patient is clearly not competent, then a hospital may be justified in detaining the patient. In *Blackman for Blackman v. Rifkin*, **the patient was extremely intoxicated and had suffered head trauma** [16]. The court ruled that the hospital was justified in restraining the patient and keeping her in the hospital because the hospital could assume that the patient would have consented to treatment if she had not been in that condition. The court dismissed her false imprisonment suit. This case must be limited to its facts. While the hospital may be justified in detaining a severely intoxicated person, the hospital cannot detain a competent patient against his or her will.

In the case of a **minor,** the hospital can attempt to get a court order to require the family to keep the child in the hospital, but any attempt to physically restrain the child or the parent in the absence of a court order exposes the hospital to liability. Basically, you can talk to a patient until he refuses to listen to you, but you cannot physically prevent him from leaving.

It does not matter how noble your motives are. Patients have a right to refuse treatment. Patients also have a right to leave the hospital when they wish (unless they have been committed through legal procedures) and to have freedom of movement. As healthcare providers, you cannot interfere with these rights without potential liability.

One other scenario may give rise to an action for false imprisonment. **When the physician has written a discharge order, the hospital cannot keep the patient until he "settles the bill."** While the patient obviously has the obligation to pay for services rendered, the hospital cannot hold him until the patient indicates how he will pay.

Intentional Infliction of Emotional Distress

To establish the tort of intentional infliction of emotional distress, the plaintiff must show that the defendant's conduct is outrageous and beyond the bounds of common decency. Insulting behavior is not enough; the actions must be egregious. One case in which the court allowed the plaintiff to proceed with his claim of intentional infliction of emotional distress is *Williams v. Payne et al.* [17]. In *Williams,* the police suspected that the plaintiff had ingested crack cocaine. Plaintiff was brought to Pontiac Osteopathic Hospital, where the sheriff asked the physician to pump plaintiff's stomach. The physician was aware that the sheriff did not have a warrant for the search.

After placing the plaintiff in four-point restraints, the physician forcefully and over the objections of plaintiff performed a gastric lavage. Thereafter, plaintiff was involuntarily catheterized. In refusing to dismiss the claims against the hospital and doctor, the court concluded that a jury could decide whether the conduct was outrageous.

Trespass to Land

The tort of trespass to land occurs when a person, without the consent of the owner, enters on another's land or causes anyone or anything to enter the land. Harm to the land is not required, but without harm to the land, courts usually award only nominal damages. Trespass to land arises most often in the home health area.

In home care, healthcare providers are guests in the patients' homes. They are there to perform necessary medical procedures and to teach, but they are still guests in the patients' homes. At any time that a patient instructs you to leave his home, you must leave; if you do not leave, you commit trespass to land. Keep in mind that the landowner is authorized to use reasonable force to remove a trespasser. Even if your motives are noble in refusing to leave the property, such as wanting to perform necessary wound care for the patient's benefit, your intent is no defense to the tort of trespass. Other potential claims for trespass to land include those against the patient who refuses to leave a facility after being discharged and against visitors in a facility who refuse to leave after visiting hours (Box 2-1).

Box 2-1 | Intentional and Quasi-Intentional Torts

Intentional tort: a civil wrongdoing that requires intentional interference with one's person, reputation, or property.

Assault: placing someone in immediate fear or apprehension of a harmful or noxious touching without consent; the person must be aware that you are about to touch him or her.

Battery: a harmful or offensive touching of another without consent or without a legally justifiable reason; without consent or absent an emergency, any touching of a patient can be a battery.

False imprisonment: the unlawful detention of a person where he is deprived of personal liberty of movement against his will and without any authority to detain. To be falsely imprisoned, a person must be confined within a specific area against his will; he must be confined by physical, chemical, or emotional means and/or by physical force or threat of physical force; and he must be aware of the confinement.

Intentional infliction of emotional distress: conduct is outrageous and beyond the bounds of common decency. Insulting behavior is not enough; the actions must be egregious.

Trespass to land: occurs when a person, without the consent of the owner, enters on another's land or causes anyone or anything to enter the land. Harm to the land is not required, but without harm, damages are usually nominal.

Quasi-intentional torts: include defamation, invasion of privacy, and breach of confidentiality. *Quasi* means "resembling"—these types of torts resemble intentional torts but are different because they are based on speech.

Defamation: a false statement or communication that a speaker knows or should know is false and that is published to third parties and damages a person's reputation. **Truth** is an absolute defense to defamation. Libel is written defamation. Slander is oral defamation.

Invasion of privacy: unjustifiable intrusion on another's right of privacy by:
1. Appropriating his or her name or likeness
2. Unreasonably interfering with his or her seclusion
3. Publishing private facts
4. Placing the person in a false light

Invasion of privacy differs from defamation. In most instances, the information is true but is information that a person wants to keep private. While defamation causes injury to reputation, invasion of privacy causes injury to feelings.

Breach of confidentiality: a legal and ethical issue. The code of ethics of allied health personnel must emphasize that healthcare professionals must safeguard patients' right to privacy by judiciously protecting confidential information.

■ Quasi-Intentional Torts

Quasi-intentional torts include defamation, invasion of privacy, and breach of confidentiality. *Quasi* means "resembling." These types of torts resemble intentional torts but are different because they are based on speech [18].

Defamation

Defamation wrongfully damages the reputation of another person. **Libel** is written defamatory statements, and **slander** is spoken defamatory statements. To be liable for defamation, you must make a defamatory statement that is published to third parties, and the speaker must have known or should have known that the statements were false.

In defining a defamatory statement, the courts have looked to whether the statement exposed the plaintiff to public hatred, contempt, ridicule, or degradation [19]. There must be proof that there was actual harm to the person's reputation.

There are, however, certain statements that are considered **defamatory per se,** such as serious allegations of sexual misconduct or criminal behavior or allegations that the plaintiff is afflicted with a loathsome disease. Historically, loathsome diseases include syphilis, gonorrhea, and leprosy. Today, allegations of hepatitis and HIV-positive status or AIDS may well be the new loathsome diseases. If these types of defamatory statements are made, then the plaintiff does not need to prove actual damage to reputation.

An example of a defamation per se case is *Schlesser v. Keck* [20]. Plaintiff was a cook and caterer who tested false-positive for syphilis when she was in the army. She sought treatment for the false-positive. Defendant was the doctor's nurse who was administering the treatments. Despite the defendant's knowledge that the tests were false-positive and the defendant's knowledge that plaintiff did not have syphilis, defendant announced at a party that the plaintiff had syphilis and should not be allowed to cater or prepare food.

In addition to making a defamatory statement, there must be publication to a third person. You cannot defame someone by telling only him or her. Finally, you must know or you should have known that the statements were false.

Defenses

Truth is an absolute defense to defamation. Even if a true statement damages a person's reputation, it is not actionable as defamation. Certain individuals, such as public officials, must prove actual malice on the part of the defendant before they are allowed to succeed.

In addition to the above, there may be **qualified privileges** that protect a person from a defamation suit. **One of the most common is the qualified privilege all states have enacted concerning the reporting of elder or child abuse.** As long as the report is made in good faith, the healthcare provider is protected from liability. Most states have also granted **peer review members** a qualified privilege. Such individuals must be members of a properly convened peer review committee; the committee must be duly authorized by the facility to conduct peer review; and the comments made in the committee meeting and all reports of the committee must be confidential. While the member of a peer review committee may have a qualified privilege to speak freely within the confines of the committee, that privilege does not extend to speaking freely about the committee findings or proceedings to individuals not involved with the peer review committee.

The greatest liability for defamation suits results from statements made about coworkers, especially when future employers seek references. Even though a qualified privilege exists to give a good-faith assessment of an employee's job performance, many businesses have opted only to verify dates of employment to avoid any allegation of defamation. **Under no circumstances should anyone give his unsolicited opinion about a former employee.**

In *Ironside v. Simi Valley Hospital,* a physician sued the hospital for sending an unsolicited letter to the physician's new employer stating that the physician had had his privileges summarily suspended and that a report to that effect had been sent to the California Medical Board [21]. The letter suggested that the new employer check the status of the physician's license to practice medicine with the California Medical Board. In actuality, there had been no suspension or limitation placed on the physician's license. The letter, however, did imply that there had been. Likewise, in *Simpkins v. District of Columbia et al.,* the court held that a plaintiff physician could proceed against defendants who allegedly reported to a physician data bank that the physician had resigned his staff privileges at the hospital during a review of the quality of care he provided [22].

Lessons learned:

- Do not talk about your fellow employees.
- If you are in a supervisory position, keep all comments about the quality of care a person renders confidential.
- All inquiries concerning former employees should be referred to one designated department in the facility to maintain standardization.
- Before any information is released about a former employee, have the employee's written consent to release the information as well as an agreement to release the facility from liability with regard to the information released.

Invasion of Privacy

Invasion of privacy is the tort of unjustifiably intruding upon another's right of privacy by:

1. Appropriating his or her name or likeness
2. Unreasonably interfering with his or her seclusion
3. Publishing private facts
4. Placing a person in a false light

Invasion of privacy differs from defamation. In most instances, the information is true but is information that a person wants to keep private. While defamation causes injury to reputation, invasion of privacy causes injury to feelings.

Appropriating Likeness and Placing Person in a False Light

In the medical setting the most common example of appropriating likeness is the use of photographs or video images of the patient without consent or exceeding the scope of the consent. For example, in *Vassiliades v. Garfinckel's, Brooks Brothers,* a plastic surgeon used before-and-after pictures of a patient in a public demonstration without the patient's consent [23]. Another example is the use of a video of a Cesarean section not for medical teaching purposes but for inclusion in a movie that was shown publicly in movie theaters [24].

If a patient gives consent to the use of his or her likeness for teaching purposes or treatment purposes, the scope of the consent cannot be exceeded. If the patient does not give consent, then no likeness can be used at all for any reason.

▪ ▪ ▪ **What If?** ────────────────

A local politician has extensive cosmetic dental work and plastic surgery performed in the hospital and clinic where you work. You tell your family, and the patient learns of this from someone in the local community. In other words, her privacy has been breached.
1. What are the legal and ethical implications?

Publicizing Private Facts

The most basic right of patients is to expect healthcare professionals to keep all information obtained in the treatment of the patient confidential. Every state mandates that the patient's confidentiality be maintained. Every state outlines only limited situations in which a person may release information concerning a patient without his consent.

In *Estate of Behringer v. Princeton Medical Center*, a successful ear, nose, and throat surgeon who practiced at the medical center was admitted for tests and diagnosed with AIDS [25]. No special steps were taken to protect the medical record or the patient's privacy. In fact, the physicians and nurses who cared for the doctor spoke openly about his condition to individuals who had no involvement in his care. By the time the doctor was discharged from the hospital, numerous persons in the community knew of his condition and his practice was adversely affected.

In holding that the physician could bring suit against the medical center for invasion of privacy, the court stated: "The information was too easily available, too titillating to disregard. All that was required was a glance at the chart, and the written words became whispers and the whispers became roars" [26]. The whispers should never have taken place.

Likewise, in *Doe v. Methodist Hospital*, a patient's HIV status was openly discussed with individuals not involved with his care [27]. Plaintiff suffered a heart attack and was taken to the hospital by paramedics. He disclosed to the paramedics his HIV status. They noted this on their report, which became part of the medical record. One of plaintiff's coworkers called his wife, who was a nurse at the hospital, and she reviewed the patient's records and told her husband the plaintiff's HIV status. While the Indiana Supreme Court ruled that Indiana does not recognize the tort of invasion of privacy, the suit was allowed to proceed under other causes of actions.

Even disclosing information to other healthcare professionals may lead to a lawsuit. In *Saur v. Probes*, plaintiff's wife attempted to have plaintiff involuntarily committed for psychiatric treatment [28]. She went to court and the court appointed a psychiatrist to examine the plaintiff. The court-appointed psychiatrist contacted the defendant, who had been plaintiff's treating physician for several months. The two physicians discussed the plaintiff's medical condition. The plaintiff filed the action against his treating psychiatrist, alleging that the psychiatrist disclosed confidential information obtained during the course of treatment without his permission. The lower court dismissed the plaintiff's case, but the higher court reversed, finding that plaintiff was entitled to have his case heard before a jury to decide whether the disclosure was appropriate. Whether this plaintiff ultimately wins is not the issue. The issue is that the court allowed the case to proceed to the jury.

Being a healthcare provider and working in a medical facility do not give you the right to unlimited access to all patients' medical records. The law allows you to view and use only the medical records of the patients you are treating.

These cases teach some important lessons. Disclosure of confidential patient information may lead to lawsuits and disciplinary actions under legal theories of liability such as:
- Breach of contract
- Breach of confidentiality
- Negligence
- Intentional infliction of emotional distress
- Defamation

Breach of Confidentiality

The computer age is creating even more problems for **breach of confidentiality.** While allowing practitioners to have easier access to their patient records and allowing information to be relayed more quickly, computerized medical records allow too many people access. A case in point was filed in 1997 in Fulton County, Georgia. In *Ruocco v. Emory Hospital*, plaintiff filed a lawsuit alleging invasion of privacy, negligent maintenance of records, negligent supervision, intentional infliction of emotional distress, and defamation [29].

Plaintiff was a nurse employed by the hospital who was taking part in a hepatitis study. She received injections as part of the study. When she missed several weeks of work, one of the doctors in the study accessed her electronic medical record without the plaintiff's permission. Although he was not plaintiff's treating physician, he accessed the records by claiming to be her physician. He was not. He did not tell the plaintiff he accessed the records and, in fact, in his deposition he stated that he never intended to tell her. Plaintiff learned of the unauthorized access when she accessed her own records and saw that someone had accessed her records without her consent. The concern over electronic access to medical records has been increasing. In 1996, Congress enacted the **Health Insurance Portability and Accountability Act of 1996 (HIPAA),** calling for regulations to establish criteria for a federal standard in authorizing the release of medical information. In February 2000 the U.S. Department of Health and Human Services published the final rules to establish the federal criteria.

Whether a healthcare provider has access to the traditional written medical record or to computerized records, the responsibility to keep information confidential does not change. **Any information that a healthcare provider learns while taking care of a patient is confidential, even if it does not relate directly to the treatment of the patient.**

The issue of confidentiality is both a legal and an ethical issue. The code of ethics of allied health personnel must emphasize that the healthcare professional must safeguard the patient's right to privacy by judiciously protecting confidential information. Many other groups, such as the Hospice Association of America, the American Nurses Association, the National League for Nursing, and the American Hospital Association, recognize as a basic right of patients the confidentiality of the assessments, treatment, and information contained in the patient's medical records.

■ Intentional and Quasi-Intentional Torts and Insurance Policies

Even though medical malpractice polices have historically covered intentional torts, many insurers are writing exclusions from coverage. This is especially true if the tort alleged involves sexual misconduct. As a healthcare provider, know what your policy covers and what it does not.

▪ ▪ ▪ What If?

An adult patient is a member of a religion that does not believe in receiving blood. The patient receives a colostomy and begins hemorrhaging. He is unable to voice his objections. You know of this patient's strong beliefs and that he does not want to receive blood. On the admission sheet, the area for religion is blank. He has no family. The nurses and doctors want to give blood and you do not want him to die.
1. What should you do?
2. What are the ethical dilemmas and legal implications if he receives blood?
3. What are the legal and ethical implications if the patient is a minor and the parents refuse blood?

▪ ▪ ▪ What If?

An Alzheimer's patient strikes you in the face and breaks your nose. You strike back to defend yourself and you injure the patient.
1. What are the ethical implications?
2. What are the legal implications?
3. Can you sue the patient for a broken nose?
4. Can you file criminal charges for assault and battery?
5. Can you file a claim for worker's compensation because you received an injury while working?
6. Can the patient sue you or file charges?
7. What are the patient's rights?

■ Conclusion

The performance of day-to-day patient care and treatment gives rise to potential liability for intentional and quasi-intentional torts. You can avoid liability if you always have your patient's consent to perform specific procedures and do not exceed that consent.

Always maintain your patient's confidentiality and speak only to those individuals who are actively involved in the patient's care. Understand that your patient has an absolute right to refuse treatment and that your ability to change a person's mind is limited to your verbal skills only. It is not true that every patient is a potential plaintiff. But a patient can become a plaintiff if you do not exercise good nursing judgment or do not have respect for your patient's rights, privacy, and freedom.

▪▪▪ Pertinent Points

1. To successfully pursue a lawsuit for an intentional tort, the plaintiff must prove that the defendant had the requisite intent, that the injury resulted from the defendant's action, and that no defense was present.
2. If a defendant can prove that the plaintiff gave consent, then the defendant did not commit an intentional tort.
3. The defendant must stay within the boundaries of the consent given by the plaintiff. If the defendant exceeds the scope of the consent, then it is as though there was no consent.
4. Forcing treatment on an unwilling patient is assault and battery.
5. If procedures for involuntary admissions are not followed, then false imprisonment may occur. If force is used to detain a patient, then false imprisonment has occurred. No matter how noble a healthcare worker's motives may be, he has no right to forcibly detain a patient who is competent and not a danger to himself or others.
6. Invasion of privacy is likely to occur in the healthcare setting if healthcare professionals do not maintain the confidentiality of patient records.
7. All patients have the right to expect that healthcare professionals will maintain the confidentiality of medical records.
8. Trespass to land occurs most often in the home health setting.

▪▪▪ Study Questions

1. Define an intentional tort and quasi-intentional tort.
2. Give examples of and discuss elements of and defenses for the following torts:
   a. Assault
   b. Battery
   c. False imprisonment
   d. Defamation

    e. Invasion of privacy

    f. Intentional infliction of emotional distress

    g. Trespass to land.

3. Discuss the intent required to commit an intentional tort.

4. Discuss the effects of consent as a defense to an intentional tort.

5. Discuss a recent case with the class involving an intentional or quasi-intentional tort in your area. (Use the recommended websites.)

6. Discuss the ethical implications of committing an intentional or quasi-intentional tort.

7. Discuss how you can protect a patient's privacy.

8. Using free legal websites, find a case based on an allegation of a lack of informed consent in your practice area.

9. Discuss potential disciplinary actions from involvement in an intentional or quasi-intentional tort.

10. Discuss how charting can prevent a successful lawsuit based on false imprisonment.

▪ ▪ ▪ References

1. Schloendorff v. Soc'y of N.Y. Hosp., 105 N.E. 92 (1914).

2. Pizzaloto v. Wilson, 437 So. 2d 859 (La. 1983).

3. Guin v. Sison, 552 So. 2d 60 (La. 1989).

4. Montgomery v. Bazaz-Shegal, 742 A.2d 1125 (Pa. 1999).

5. Roberson v. Provident House, 576 So. 2d 992 (La. 1991).

6. O'Brien v. Cunard S.S. Co., 28 N.E. 266 (1881).

7. Novak v. Cobb County Kennestone Hosp. Auth., No. 94–8403, slip. op. (11th Cir. 1996).

8. DiLeo v. Nugent, 592 A.2d 1126 (Md. 1991).

9. Smith v. St. Paul Fire and Marine Ins. Co., 353 N.W.2d 130 (Minn. 1984).

10. St. Paul Fire and Marine Ins. Co. v. Asbury, 720 P.3d 540 (Ariz. 1986).

11. St. Paul Fire and Marine Ins. Co. v. Shernow, 610 A.2d 1281 (Conn. 1992).

12. Brand v. Univ. Hosp., 525 S.E.2d 374 (Ga. 1999).

13. Mawhirt v. Ahmed, 86 F.Supp.2d 81 (E.D.N.Y. 2000).

14. Davis v. St. Jude Med. Ctr., 645 So. 2d 771 (La. App. 5th Cir. 1994).

15. Big Town Nursing Home, Inc. v. New, 461 S.W.2d 195 (Tex. 1970).

16. Blackman for Blackman v. Rifkin, 759 P.2d 54 (Colo. 1988).

17. Williams v. Payne et al., 73 F. Supp. 2d 785 (E.D. Mich. 1999).

18. Aiken T. (Ed.) (2004). *Legal, Ethical, and Political Issues in Nursing* (2nd ed). Philadelphia: F.A. Davis Company.

19. Phipps v. Clark Oil and Ref. Corp., 408 N.W.2d 569, 573 (Minn. 1987).

20. Schlesser v. Keck, 271 P.2d 588 (Cal. 1954).

21. Ironside v. Simi Valley Hosp., No. 95–6336, slip op. (6th Cir. 1996).

22. Simpkins v. District of Columbia et al., No. 94-5243, slip op. (D.C. Cir. 1997).
23. Vassiliades v. Garfinckel's, Brooks Bros., 492 A.2d 580 (D.C. 1985).
24. Feeney v. Young, 191 A.D. 501, 181 N.Y. Supp. 481 (1920).
25. Estate of Behringer v. Princeton Med. Ctr., 592 A.2d 1251 (N.J. 1991).
26. *Id.* at 1273.
27. Doe v. Methodist Hosp., 639 N.E.2d 683 (Ind. 1994, *rev'd*, 690 N.E.2d 681 (Ind. 1997).
28. Saur v. Probes, 476 N.W.2d 496 (Mich. 1991).
29. Ruocco v. Emory Hosp., no. 97-VS0132401.

▪ ▪ ▪ Resources

Law Library of Congress, www.loc.gov.

Professional Liability Insurance

3

Key Chapter Concepts

- Aggregate Limit
- Claims-Made Policy
- "Dec" Page
- Disciplinary Defense Insurance
- Endorsement
- Excess Coverage
- Exclusions
- Indemnification
- Insuring Agreement or Clause
- Occurrence Basis Policy
- Policy Jacket
- Premium
- Prior Acts Coverage
- Self-insurance
- Tail Coverage
- Umbrella Coverage

Objectives

At the conclusion of this chapter, the reader will be able to:

1. Define the basic professional liability insurance terms, concepts, and types of policies.
2. Discuss the necessity for professional liability insurance for independent contractors and employed healthcare professionals.
3. Discuss the employer's liability policy exclusions and their effect on individual employee liability.
4. Outline the typical components of a professional liability policy.
5. Discuss what is covered in a disciplinary defense insurance policy.

■ Liability Insurance in General

The overall purpose of liability insurance is to spread the risk of economic loss among members of a group who have a commonly shared risk. A small fee, a **premium,** is paid by each insured member and pooled by the insurer into a fund. The insurer then uses this fund to pay for claims against any of the members. This avoids the often economically devastating costs associated with defending yourself against such claims. Nonmeritorious claims can be just as costly to defend as meritorious ones.

Case Scenario

A patient was treated as an outpatient at a medical facility and prescribed a sulfa drug. The patient was allergic to sulfa drugs, a fact that was noted in the written medical record. However, the medical records technician did not transcribe the allergy note into the computerized patient record. Upon discharge from the facility, the nurse failed to check the written record. The pharmacist who dispensed the drug did not note the allergy. After taking one dose of the sulfa drug, the patient had a severe allergic reaction that ultimately led to her death. The patient's family sued the pharmacist and the facility for the negligence of the nurse and the medical records technician. If the claim against the technician was made after the technician left the facility's employ, did the facility's liability insurance provide coverage to defend the technician? You will learn the answer at the end of this chapter.

Individually, the primary objective is to protect your assets in the event of a judgment or settlement in favor of the claimant. Some professionals do not see a need to obtain liability insurance either because they believe that they do not have that much to protect or because their employers tell them that having their own insurance makes them targets and more likely to be sued. They believe they are "judgment free," so that even if a claim against them is successful, they have little that the claimant could collect. This assumption is erroneous. First, although a person has few assets now, it is reasonable to assume that most professionals will have assets worth protecting in the future. If a claimant secures a judgment against you, that judgment stands and can be enforced at a later time, when your assets may have increased substantially. Even if you have insurance by that time, it will not provide coverage. Besides losing a substantial portion of your assets, there may be worse ramifications, such as bankruptcy.

■ Independent Contractors and Employed Professionals: The Need for an Individual Policy

A healthcare professional who is an independent contractor most definitely should obtain liability insurance. An **independent contractor** is a person who is self-employed and who enters into contracts to provide professional services to various entities such as medical facilities, doctors' offices, and/or individual clients. In general, these entities have no liability for the acts or omissions of an independent contractor unless the entity can be found directly liable, as discussed in the next section [1]. Most of these contracting entities will require that the independent contractor show evidence of current liability coverage. Even if it is not required, securing coverage to protect your assets is exceedingly important.

The employed practitioner, even though provided coverage by the employer, should also obtain a professional liability policy. To understand why this is so, first consider employers' liability policies.

■ Employers' Liability Policies

An employer such as a hospital or doctor's office obtains professional liability insurance to protect its own interests. With respect to its liability for the negligent acts of an employee or independent contractor, the employer seeks to protect itself against claims that fall generally under two theories of liability. First, the employer can have a claim filed against it charging that it is directly liable for the injury of the claimant caused by an employee or independent contractor. Under this theory, the claimant commonly alleges the following:

1. When the employer hired the employee, the employer failed its duty to ascertain that the employee had the necessary qualifications and capability to render safe care.
2. The employer failed to perform a background check.
3. The employer failed to adequately supervise the employee.
4. The employer failed to provide the employee with the proper training required to render safe care or failed to properly assess that the employee required additional training.

The employer can also be sued under a theory of **vicarious liability,** wherein the acts or omissions of the employee are imputed to the employer, so that the employer can be found liable for them [2, 3]. (See also the legal theory called **respondeat superior**.)

Coverage and Exclusions

In general, the liability policies that employers obtain to protect themselves in the event of such allegations provide protection for the employee as well. The employer's policy spells out specifically those acts of the employee that are covered and those that are excluded from coverage. Commonly, the employee is covered under the employer's policy for a negligent act only if it was performed within the course of employment and within the scope of the employee's duties.

Acts that often are specifically excluded are those such as the **quasi-intentional torts of libel** or **slander** and **intentional acts, such as assault and battery.** If a claim is made against an employer for the acts of an employee that are covered by the policy, then the insurer has a duty to defend the employee as well as the employer. The insurer's duty to defend generally includes, for example, providing legal counsel to represent the employer and employee in negotiations, mediations, or arbitrations with the claimant; representation in court proceedings; filing court documents; investigating the alleged incident; and advising the client regarding case strategy. However, see the discussion below regarding conflicts of interest between employer and employee that can arise in such situations.

■ Self-Insurance

Some healthcare institutions elect to **self-insure** in accordance with state laws. No insurance policy is required, but an employer must provide evidence that it has sufficient funds set aside to satisfy a successful claim. Whether the employer self-insures or purchases coverage, keep in mind that the employer is looking out for the employer's own interests first and foremost. This is particularly true, however, where the employer self-insures, because then the employer has more control in the defense of a claim.

■ Employed Professionals: The Need for Their Own Professional Liability Insurance

There are a host of reasons why the prudent employed professional obtains individual professional liability insurance. The reasons for insurance are discussed in the following sections.

Acts Not Covered

The employer's policy does not provide coverage for certain acts of the employee. For example, a medical assistant makes a remark to a coworker about a client that the client overhears and reasonably perceives to be defamatory. The employer's policy will probably not provide coverage for this incident, and the employee will have to defend against a lawsuit. Even if the employee successfully defends against such allegations, the costs of doing so can be substantial. Policies are available to individuals that provide coverage for many acts that are not covered under an employer's policy.

Limits of Policy Exceeded

An employer's policy, as with any insurance policy, has limits as to how much the insurer pays. If an incident involves multiple alleged acts of negligence and/or claimants, it is possible that the employer's policy limits are exceeded. In that case, the employee may be responsible for financing all or part of the defense.

Mergers and Closures of Physicians' Offices and Healthcare Facilities

In today's healthcare environment, the "urge to merge" has resulted in complex restructuring schemes. The terms of agreement between two merging entities can result in changes in the employer's liability insurance coverage. Depending on the terms of the employer's policy and the date of an incident involving the employees, employees may find they are without employer coverage for a given incident that was covered under their employer's policy prior to the merger. A worse scenario can occur when a facility closes. The employer may not have purchased a policy to cover claims made after the closure, and the employee may therefore be left "bare," meaning that the insurance company will not pay for defense costs or money awards.

Conflict Between Employer and Employee over Respective Positions Regarding an Incident

In any given incident that results in a claim, the employer may not agree with the employee's view of that incident. For example, the employer takes the position that in a given incident the employee was not acting within the scope of his duties. If the employer proves this is true, the employer's insurer (or especially the employer if self-insured) has no duty to assist in the employee's defense [4]. At the very least, the fact that the employee and the employer disagree as to the facts of an incident can create problems in the defense strategy of the insurer's attorney. It is far better to have your own policy and your own attorney whose loyalty will be only to you, the employee.

Disagreement Between Employer and Employee over Proposed Settlements

The employer may wish to settle a claim rather than defend a lawsuit for any number of reasons; for example, the employer may wish to limit unfavorable publicity or it may not want to devote the personnel time and other resources necessary to defend the case. The employer's insurer may settle the claim if the claimant appears to have at least a 50 percent chance of winning at trial. It may be more cost effective for the insurer to settle the case rather than risk going to trial and have a judge or jury award a substantially higher amount. Even though an employee may have strong feelings about the lack of negligence on her part in an incident, the best interests of the employee are not primary; those of the employer are. If the employer is self-insured, the focus of loyalty is obvious [5].

Conflict Between Multiple Employees over an Incident

Many incidents involve multiple employees. In such situations, the claimant sues everyone connected with the incident: the employer, the supervisors, and the employees. Attorneys do not want the clients to later accuse them of negligent handling of their cases. The potential for disagreement regarding essential facts of an incident can put an individual at odds not only with supervisors but also with coworkers, who, after all, are trying to protect themselves. Your own insurer and attorney have loyalty only to you and will formulate a defense strategy that is in your best interest rather than one that must take into account the positions of all your coworkers.

Cost

A professional liability policy for an employed healthcare professional is generally inexpensive. For such a low cost and the protection that the policy affords, professionals should not practice without such a policy. Many policies also provide **disciplinary defense insurance** to pay for healthcare providers who must defend a disciplinary action before a state regulatory board in an administrative hearing (check your policy). The policy routinely covers costs of having qualified attorneys represent clients. The policy also covers:

1. Legal fee reimbursement/attorney fees
2. Reimbursement for loss of wages
3. Reimbursement for travel, food, and lodging

Peace of Mind

The benefit of knowing that you have someone on your side if you are ever involved in a claim against you is priceless. The insurer provides an attorney to assist you in your defense. Also, if a judgment is awarded against you, the insurance company pays the money award to the plaintiff. It will not come out of your pocket.

■ Applying for Professional Liability Insurance

An insurer will take into account an individual practitioner's situation in recommending policy provisions and limits of coverage. An applicant must be thorough and honest in providing information to the insurance representative. If you are an independent contractor, inform the representative of the details of your practice including, but not limited to, the following:

1. **What services do you provide?** Inform the representative in writing about your typical day-to-day duties, those services that you provide on rare occasions, as well as those that you do not provide now but are considering in the future. This prevents denial of coverage by your insurer due to your concealment or misrepresentation if an incident occurs while performing a service you did not previously mention [6]. Also, the representative will take your specific occupation into account. For example, some services provided by a physical therapist have a higher incidence of related claims than most of those provided by a medical records technician.
2. **What types of clients do you serve?** For example, are the clients frail, elderly, children, or disabled?
3. **Do you employ or supervise others, even if only occasionally?**
4. **Are you supervised and by whom?** Supervision may affect the independent contractor status.
5. **Are you in compliance with all licensing requirements, if required in your state?**

6. **Have you ever had a lawsuit or disciplinary action filed against you?**
7. **Are there any incidents that have occurred in the past that could possibly give rise to a future claim?**
8. **Did the incident occur during the course and scope of employment?**

■ Components of a Typical Professional Liability Policy

A practitioner's liability insurance policy is tailored to fit a specific type of practice (Box 3-1). However, the provisions typically include the elements discussed subsequently.

At the beginning of the policy form, there is usually a statement that it is a **claims-made** or an **occurrence basis** policy. A **claims-made trigger** means that coverage is provided for any claim made while the policy is in force.

For example, you purchase a **claims-made policy** with coverage from March 1, 2007, through March 1, 2008, but at the end of that term you decide not to renew because you are no longer going to work. If a claim is made against you on March 1, 2008, coverage applies. However, if the incident giving rise to the claim occurred during the policy period on March 1, 2007, but the claim was not made against you until June 1, 2008, there is usually no coverage unless you have tail coverage.

Some policies provide that if you notify your insurer before the expiration of the policy of an incident that you believe could evolve into a claim, then coverage is provided. Also, many

Box 3-1 | Types of Policies

- **Claims-made:** A type of professional liability insurance policy that covers injuries/damages only if the injury occurs in the policy period and only if the claim is reported or filed to the insurance company during the policy period or during the tail.
- **Occurrence basis:** Professional liability insurance policy that covers injuries/damages that occur during the period covered by the policy even though the claim may be reported or filed outside the policy period.
- **Tail coverage:** An uninterrupted extension of the insurance policy period, also known as the **extended reporting endorsement.**
- **Umbrella coverage:** Coverage purchased in addition to a basic liability policy that provides additional amount limits and/or adds coverage for events not covered in the basic policy.

policies provide, at no extra charge, a **60-day extension** following expiration of the policy during which the insurer will defend you in a claim filed during that 60-day period. If neither of these two modifications for coverage exists, then you should consider purchasing **tail coverage.** (Insurers should check the applicable statutes of limitations for filing lawsuits in their states.)

Tail Coverage

Tail coverage is a special policy that extends the coverage provided in the original policy for an agreed-on period. If in the above example you purchased a tail to extend coverage until March 1, 2009, and a claim was made on October 26, 2008, coverage applies.

Prior Acts Coverage

Another concern with claims-made policies is that they generally do not cover **prior acts,** those incidents that occurred before the beginning effective date of the policy. Prior acts coverage can be purchased for an additional premium. The insurer issues **prior acts** coverage going back for a certain period of time. The insurer requires that the professional provide the following information:
1. Services that were provided
2. Whether the professional was employed or self-employed
3. Details regarding any incident that the professional believes might possibly evolve into a claim
   Not divulging such information can result in the insurer having no obligation to provide a defense for any claim related to the nondivulged incident.

Occurrence Basis Policy

An **occurrence basis** policy provides coverage for an incident that occurs during the policy period, regardless of when the claim is made. For example, you purchase an occurrence basis policy with coverage from March 1, 2007, through March 1, 2008, but then decide not to renew the policy. If a claim is made on July 4, 2008, based on an incident that occurred during the policy period, coverage applies. You would not, however, have coverage for any incident that occurred before the beginning effective date of the policy unless you purchased prior acts coverage.
   Occurrence basis coverage offers the safest protection because you usually know whether an incident will trigger a claim. Insurers

are increasingly omitting occurrence policies in favor of **claims-made policies.** This is probably because the period of time for which an insurer must be concerned about a claim can be definitely determined.

Medical facilities usually obtain occurrence policies [7]. Under such a policy, if you no longer work for the employer, the employer and you still have coverage for an incident that occurred while you were employed. However, if the employer has a claims-made policy, then your coverage depends on the policy provisions. The importance of knowing the provisions in your employer's policy is evident because you should know whether to consider purchasing **tail coverage.**

Declarations Page

The declarations page, frequently called the **"dec page"** in insurance jargon, is where the policy lists the name(s) of the person or institution insured. The **aggregate limit** is the total amount that the insurer pays during the policy period, usually one year, regardless of the number of incidents, claims, claimants, or defendants. For example, the employer's policy dec page provides for $3 million of aggregate coverage.

Assume that the incident described in the previous example has occurred and that $1 million has been used to provide a defense for that incident. Then $2 million of coverage remains for the balance of the policy period. This may seem like a large amount, but it can easily be exhausted if the institution has several serious incidents that occur during a policy period, and it provides another reason why you should consider obtaining a personal policy.

The dec page also notes the dates indicating the period of time for which coverage is provided and the premium charged.

In the case of an employer, it also lists the categories of employees who are covered. In addition, the dec page will spell out the **limitations of liability.**

There are two types of limitations on liability: **per incident** or **occurrence** and **aggregate,** and there are dollar amounts noted for each type. **Per incident** (in a health professional's policy it is usually called a **medical incident**) amounts show the maximum amount that the insurer will pay to defend a claim that arises from a single incident.

For example, the dec page shows "$1,000,000 per incident." This means that the insurer pays up to that amount only, regardless of the number of claimants or insured involved. Suppose that three radiology technicians are negligent in transferring a patient from the X-ray table to the gurney and the patient falls, sustaining a serious head injury. The patient sues for the injury. The spouse sues for loss of consortium, and the patient's child sues for loss of society and companionship. An employer's policy having $1 million per incident coverage pays for the defense of the employer. This amount is also used to pay for the defense of the radiology technicians. This illustrates once more the importance of healthcare employees purchasing their own liability policies.

The practitioner may also want to consider additional liability protection by purchasing an **umbrella policy.** The maximum amount payable under a basic liability policy may become exhausted, for example, when there are multiple claims. An umbrella policy provides coverage beyond the amount limits of the basic policy. It may also provide coverage for events excluded from coverage under a basic policy. For example, an umbrella policy may be written to provide coverage for allegations of defamation where there is no such coverage under the basic policy. The amount of coverage desired and the particular events covered determine the cost of an umbrella policy. The practitioner should discuss his or her particular situation with an insurance representative to determine whether the addition of an umbrella policy is appropriate.

■ Additional Coverage

Insurance companies that provide professional liability insurance may also provide additional coverage, including the following:
1. **Defendant expense benefit:** reimburses aggregate wages up to a limit and covered expenses incurred when a healthcare provider is on trial as a defendant in a claim covered by insurance.
2. **License protection:** reimburses up to a limit for defense or disciplinary actions or other covered expenses arising out of an incident covered.
3. **Personal liability protection:** covers up to limits chosen for liability damages for covered claims unrelated to work resulting from incidents at your personal residence.
4. **Medical payments:** pays up to the amount determined and reimburses medical expenses to persons injured at your premises or home.
5. **Assault coverage:** covers medical expenses or property damage and reimburses up to a specific amount per incident if you are assaulted at work or while commuting to and from the workplace.

6. **Personal injury protection:** protects you up to specified limits against claims of slander, assault, battery, and privacy violation, or other alleged personal injuries committed in the provision of professional services.
7. **First aid benefit:** reimburses up to a specified amount for expenses incurred from rendering first aid to others.
8. **Damage to property of others:** pays up to a specified aggregate amount for damage incidents you accidentally cause to others' property.
9. **Deposition representation:** reimburses up to a specified amount for attorneys' fees for depositions required for incidences arising out of professional services.

■ Individual Professional Liability Policies

Regarding individual professional liability policies, most practitioners obtain policies with limits of $1 million per medical incident and $3 million in aggregate. However, insurers offer higher limits, and practitioners should discuss their particular practices with a representative to determine what coverage level is appropriate.

■ Policy Provisions

The **policy jacket** is the section that sets forth the generic provisions found in most policies of the same type (Box 3-2). The provisions are usually separated into separate sections and generally include the elements discussed in the subsequent sections.

Box 3-2 | Policy Provisions

- Statement of agreement
- Exclusions
- Duties and cooperation of insured
- Definitions
- Nonrenewal or cancellation
- Right to defend or settle
- Other insurance

Statement of the Agreement

This statement is often called the **insuring agreement** or **insuring clause** and states the agreement between the insurer and the insured as to what coverage is provided. The clause briefly states what types of claims (e.g., damages due to injury) the insurer is obligated to pay and under what conditions (e.g., injury due to acts or omissions of the insured) while the policy is in force.

Exclusions

The exclusions section details all the circumstances for which coverage is provided. Typical examples include, but are not limited to, claims
1. Alleging defamation or discrimination
2. Resulting from an incident that occurred before the effective date of the policy
3. Resulting from an injury the insured either expected or intended
4. Arising under any contract the insured has wherein the insured agreed to assume the liability of others
5. Arising out of the commission of a criminal act
6. Arising out of sexual misconduct with a patient or sexual assault

Duties and Cooperation of Insured

The duties and cooperation section lists the duties and required cooperation of the insured in the event of a claim and/or incident. It states how soon after a claim the insured must notify the insurer. Sometimes this is a specific number of days, but commonly the time frame may be quite vague, saying "as soon as practicable." There may or may not be a requirement that the notification be in writing. However, the prudent professional sends written notification by certified mail with a return receipt requested. The cooperation of the insured usually includes assistance in securing and giving evidence, attendance at hearings and trials, help securing the attendance of witnesses, and assistance in enforcing any right of "contribution" or "indemnity" that the insured has against others.

A right of **contribution** arises when there are others who, though not named in a claim, bear at least some responsibility for the incident. The insured, if found liable, has a right in some states to seek contribution from others based on a percentage of their responsibility in causing the incident. A right to **indemnification** arises under similar circumstances, except the insured contends that some other person was totally responsible for the incident and that other person should reimburse the insured for the entire amount he or she has paid [8].

▪ ▪ ▪ What If?

You have a medical malpractice suit filed against you. You did not have professional liability insurance. You decide to get insurance and where the forms ask, "Do you have any potential claims that may be filed?" you answer no.

1. What are the ethical implications?
2. What are the legal issues of falsifying a document?

Definitions

All of the words in a policy that are considered insurance terms that the average person may not know are defined in the policy jacket. Also defined are those terms that the insurer wants to be sure that the courts will construe in a certain way if a question of coverage arises. Such words as *medical incidents, claim, injury,* and even *you* are usually defined.

Nonrenewal or Cancellation

The nonrenewal or cancellation section describes the conditions under which the insurer can elect to not renew or to cancel the policy. Usually, the insurer does not need to have a reason. However, there are generally requirements for providing notice to the insured. Typically, if the insurer is not renewing the policy, it must notify the insured in writing at least 30 days before the policy expiration date. If the insurer plans to cancel the policy, most policy provisions state that it must provide written notice at least 10 days before cancellation for nonpayment of the premium and at least 30 days before cancellation if for any other reason.

Right to Defend or Settle

The insurer states in this right to defend or settle section its duty to defend claims as well as its right to do so, even if the facts indicate that the claim has no merit or appears to be fraudulent [9]. This is the section where the insurer may also state that it has a right to settle a claim, if it determines that settlement is appropriate, without the permission of the insured. One reason the insurer may offer settlement to a claimant is that it believes the claimant has a plausible claim that may result in a high jury award if litigated. Also, the claimant may offer to settle for an amount that the insurer believes is less than the claimant might receive if he or she prevails at trial. In either case, the insured may have little or no input in the decision, even if the insured believes that he or she has done nothing wrong.

Other Insurance

Typically, the other insurance section addresses how the payment of claims is affected if there is other insurance available to pay a given claim. This situation arises when, for example, an employer's policy and a second (e.g., professional's individual) policy provide coverage for a single medical incident. The employer's policy may state that it will only apply coverage after the second policy's limits have been paid. The amount the insurer is obligated to pay after the second policy has been paid is called **excess coverage.** If the second policy has the same provision, so that both policies are excess coverage, then the two insurers will generally share equally in the total amount paid to defend the claim [10].

Expenses of Defending a Claim

Some policies provide that the expenses (e.g., attorneys' fees, expert witness fees) are included in the limits of liability amounts. This reduces the amount available to pay the claimant's damages, regardless of whether the damages are determined by settlement, mediation, or arbitration. Other policies provide that expenses are paid over and above whatever the claimant actually receives.

Premium Payments

Usually, the premium section does not provide information regarding the time, method, or amount of the premium but states that the rates are in accordance with those in effect at the time and that the premiums are payable when they become due. As discussed earlier, an insurer generally cannot cancel a policy for default in premium payment until it has provided to the insured a timely notice of premium due and intent to cancel before cancellation.

Endorsements

The policy usually contains added provisions that delete or modify the coverage provided in the standard provisions or policy jacket of the policy. These provisions, sometimes called **riders,** address items that apply to the insured's specific situation. For example, there may be a provision that the insurer pays for expenses resulting from the insured being the victim of an assault while at work or possibly while traveling to and from work. The insurer may provide coverage for claims based on defamation or other nonmedical incidents. The insurer may grant an option to the insured to extend liability coverage (i.e., to purchase tail coverage) upon termination of the policy.

■ Before Purchasing a Policy

The time to determine what protection a professional liability policy provides is before its purchase, not when a claim is filed. Before purchase, a professional should obtain a sample policy and discuss any questions with the insurance agent. When the policy is issued, the professional should read the entire policy to be sure that it provides the coverage discussed with the agent. Even the most proficient and careful practitioners can be sued when there is no wrongful act or neglect on their part. Having a liability policy ensures that professionals are not subject to the possible economic disaster than can result in defending a claim or having a judgment awarded against them.

■ Conclusion

Let us return to the case scenario at the beginning of this chapter, which is based on a similar set of facts in a real case where the medical records technician was, indeed, sued [11]. As you learned in this chapter, whether the employer's liability policy provides a defense for the technician depends on the type of policy the employer has. If it is an occurrence basis policy, then the technician is covered, even though the technician is no longer employed at the facility, because the incident occurred during the policy period. However, if it is a claims-made policy, then coverage depends on whether there are any policy provisions that allow coverage. If the technician wisely obtained an individual policy, taking into account the possible need for tail coverage, then the professional has coverage.

■ ■ ■ **Pertinent Points**

1. Healthcare professionals should obtain their own professional liability insurance whether they are practicing as an independent contractor or as an employee of a facility.
2. Healthcare professionals should have a comprehensive understanding of all aspects of a professional liability policy before they purchase it, including whether disciplinary defense insurance, costs, and attorneys' fees are provided for in the policy.
3. Healthcare employees should be knowledgeable of the provisions in their employer's liability policy.
4. The exclusions in an employer's liability policy can result in no coverage for specific incidents involving employees or can give rise to conflicts of interest between employer and employee.
5. There are two types of professional liability insurance policies: claims-made and occurrence basis.
6. A tail may be purchased to extend coverage.

■ ■ ■ **Study Questions**

1. What is the purpose of professional liability insurance?
2. How does an independent contractor differ from an employee?
3. What is vicarious liability?
4. How is employers' self-insurance different from when they buy an insurance policy?
5. Why do you, as a healthcare professional, need professional liability insurance? List and discuss nine reasons.
6. List and discuss the topics that independent contractors should discuss with an insurance representative when applying for professional liability insurance.
7. What are the components of a typical professional liability policy? List and discuss them.
8. How does a claims-made policy differ from an occurrence basis policy?
9. Discuss the typical policy provisions found in individual professional policies.
10. What should you do before purchasing a professional liability policy?
11. Search the Internet and find two companies writing policies for your area of practice.
12. Search the Internet or discuss disciplinary actions that have been taken against healthcare providers in your field.

13. Discuss why you should have disciplinary defense insurance.
14. Define independent contractor.
15. Search the Internet and discuss a case based on medical malpractice in your field.

■ ■ ■ References

1. Prosser, W. (1971). *Handbook of the Law of Torts* (pp. 468–475). St. Paul: West Publishing Co.
2. *Id.* at 458–59.
3. Smith, J. W. (1998). *Hospital Liability* (§ 5.01(7)). New York: Law Journal Seminars-Press.
4. Glannon, J. W. (1995). *The Law of Torts* (pp. 375–378). Boston: Little, Brown & Co.
5. Smith, *supra* note 3, at § 5.02(3).
6. Dobbyn, J. F. (1989). *Insurance Law* (pp. 152–160). St. Paul: West Publishing Co.
7. Smith, *supra* note 3, at § 5.01(3).
8. Prosser, *supra* note 1, at 305–313.
9. Smith, *supra* note 3, at § 5.01(6).
10. *Id.* at § 5.01(7).
11. Harris County Hosp. Dist. v. Estrada, 872 S.W.2d 729 (Tex. 1993).

■ ■ ■ Resources

Aiken, TD. (2004). Chapter 16: Professional Liability Insurance. In: Legal, Ethical, and Political Issues in Nursing. (2nd ed.). Philadelphia: F.A. Davis Company.

www.NurseLaw.com—Nurse Attorney Institute

4

Informed Consent Issues

Key Chapter Concepts

- Battery
- Competency
- Do-Not-Resuscitate Order
- Healthcare Proxy
- Informed Consent
- Living Will
- Medical Durable Power of Attorney
- Minor
- Negligence
- Surrogate Decision Maker
- Therapeutic Privilege Exception

Objectives

At the conclusion of this chapter, the reader will be able to:

1. Define the healthcare worker's obligations regarding the informed consent process.
2. Discuss who may give consent on behalf of the patient when the patient is unable to do so.
3. Discuss what kinds of circumstances may give rise to special rules regarding informed consent.

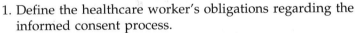

■ Battery and Negligence

The law regarding informed consent has been evolving since the early part of the twentieth century. In 1914, Justice Cardozo made the now-famous statement quoted in Box 4-1 [1]. This statement has served as the foundation for the principles of informed consent

Box 4-1 | Foundation for Informed Consent Doctrine

"Every human being of adult years and sound mind has the right to determine what shall be done with his own body."

Justice Cardozo

as we know them today. Following this case, the law defined unwanted or unauthorized medical treatment as a battery. A battery occurs whenever one person intentionally touches another without permission. Theoretically, a claim for battery arises if the patient consents to a particular procedure and the physician goes beyond the scope of that consent. A battery also occurs if a physician or healthcare provider performs a different procedure for which he or she did not obtain consent.

As the law regarding informed consent began to develop, courts slowly moved away from classifying lack of informed consent as a battery. Instead, courts have ruled that informed consent more properly belongs in the area of negligence law, the classification of medical malpractice. In the leading case of *Cobbs v. Grant* [2], the California Supreme Court explained that battery should be reserved for those circumstances where no consent at all had been obtained. Where the issue is failure to disclose a particular risk, the lawsuit is more appropriately one for negligence.

As courts across the country began to rule on battery and negligence cases, the concept of informed consent became more defined. The individual's fundamental right to control what happens to his or her body cannot be taken away except in exceptional circumstances. This right includes the right to decide whether to accept or reject proposed medical treatment. The healthcare provider has both a legal and an ethical obligation to obtain the patient's consent or the consent of the patient's legal representative before performing any kind of significant medical treatment (Boxes 4-2 and 4-3).

Case Scenario

Mrs. Richards is an elderly woman who is in the advanced stages of Alzheimer's disease. Her husband has been noticing that lately she has had bloody stools. On Tuesday, Mrs. Richards comes to the hospital for a colonoscopy procedure to rule out colon cancer. Susan White is the radiology technician working in the radiology department that day. When

Mrs. Richards arrives with her husband, Susan escorts them into a waiting area. Susan notes that the consent form for the procedure has not been signed. Susan hands the form to Mrs. Richards and asks her to sign it. Mr. Richards takes the form out of her hands and says that he has always made the decisions in their family and that he is going to sign the form. He then proceeds to ask Susan to explain the potential risks and side effects of the procedure. She attempts to answer his questions as best she can. Susan is uncertain whether Mr. Richards should sign the consent form, but she lets him do it. The principles of informed consent discussed in this chapter will help us analyze Susan's dilemma.

Box 4-2 | Elements of Disclosure for Informed Consent

1. Name of person or persons providing treatment or procedure
2. Diagnosis or suspected diagnosis of the patient/client
3. Conflicts of interest
4. Nature and purpose of the proposed procedure or treatment
5. Material risks, side effects, complications, and consequences of the proposed procedure or treatment
6. Benefits and anticipated outcome of the proposed procedure or treatment
7. Available alternatives of treatment and procedure, if any
8. Consequences of no treatment

Box 4-3 | Exceptions to Informed Consent

1. Emergency situations
2. Waiver of the right to receive information from the healthcare provider
3. Medical judgment that information would be harmful to the patient or the patient would not receive lifesaving treatment (therapeutic privilege)
4. Obvious risk
5. Public health requirement

■ Obligation to Obtain Informed Consent

The obligation to obtain informed consent ordinarily resides with the physician or healthcare provider who is performing the procedure or treatment. For example, the physician should be the one to explain to the patient the material risks and benefits of a proposed surgery. When other healthcare providers with independent authority will perform the procedure, such as a nurse-practitioner or physician's assistant, the duty to obtain informed consent may fall upon those individuals. Whenever a physician will perform or oversee the procedure, the primary responsibility for obtaining informed consent falls upon the physician even though there may be other people involved in the care. For example, when a procedure involves others (e.g., technicians or nurses), these individuals should not take it upon themselves to explain the material risks and benefits of the procedure to the patient. However, the nurse or technician should bring problems and misunderstandings to the attention of the physician or a supervisor. Furthermore, the nurse or technician may serve as a witness when the patient signs the consent form. Most healthcare facilities have specific policies relating to informed consent obligations. You should become familiar with your employer's rules regarding the informed consent process. Cases typically filed involve claims for medical malpractice and medical battery based on a lack of informed consent. A medical battery is an unpermitted "touching" of a patient. For example, a patient signs an informed consent for amputation of the right leg; however, the left leg is removed. The unpermitted "touching" or amputation of the left leg is a medical battery.

■ Disclosure Requirements

Before performing medical treatment, the physician has the duty to disclose to the patient enough information to enable the patient to make an informed decision about whether to accept or reject the treatment (see Box 4-2). Courts have generally agreed that the patient must be advised about the nature and purpose of the treatment, the material risks and consequences of the treatment, the alternative courses of treatment, and the consequences of refusing the recommended treatment. The physician should explain the type of treatment involved and the kinds of results that are being sought. Failure to explain to the patient the material risks of a treatment or procedure or the extent of the risks involved is the most common source of liability for lack of informed consent. Ordinarily, the physician is expected to disclose the most frequently experienced side effects of the proposed treatment, as well as the most significant ones. The physician should also explain the anticipated consequences for refusing to undergo the recommended treatment. (For example, refusal to undergo a rectal exam or a colonoscopy may result in the inability to detect colon cancer.) To obtain true consent, the patient must be given the opportunity to evaluate all the options available. To do so, the patient must also be told all the risks associated with each option.

The difficult question becomes how detailed to make the description of the risks and consequences. Some procedures are so simple and their risks so minor that informed consent is usually not obtained for them. For example, the risk of bruising and pain from a phlebotomy procedure (withdrawing blood from a vein) are common knowledge and usually not explained to the patient every time blood is drawn. However, more complicated procedures may carry significant risks. These risks are usually beyond the everyday knowledge of ordinary people. The physician should explain the risks of any kind of surgery because these risks are likely to be outside the knowledge of the ordinary individual. The physician should also disclose all risks that may be material and important to the patient's decision. In the case of *Canterbury v. Spence* [3], the physician failed to inform the young patient's mother of the risk of paralysis associated with surgery to remove part of the patient's vertebrae. The court ruled that the physician violated his duty to disclose the significant dangers lurking in the proposed treatment when the mother consented to the surgery.

In addition to disclosing the known risks of a proposed treatment, the physician must also explain to the patient the consequences of refusing the treatment. In the case of *Truman v. Thomas* [4], the physician failed to inform the patient of the material risks of refusing recommended Pap smears between the years 1964 and 1969. The patient was diagnosed with cancer of the cervix in 1969 and died in 1970. The court ruled that the physician breached his duty to the patient by failing to inform her of the potentially fatal consequences of allowing cervical cancer to develop undetected by a Pap smear. This case is a prime example of what has become known as the concept of **informed refusal** of treatment. The physician must disclose both the risks of the recommended treatment and the potential consequences of refusing the treatment.

The laws around the country have viewed the physician's duty to disclose material risks of a proposed treatment in two different ways: **(1) from the physician's perspective or (2) from the patient's perspective.** In most states, the physician's duty to disclose information is judged against what other physicians would disclose in similar circumstances. Under this standard, the informed consent obligation is viewed from the perspective of the physician: What would a reasonable physician ordinarily think is important enough to warn the patient regarding his case? For example, if most physicians ordinarily tell their patients about a particular side effect of a drug, the physician would be faulted for not disclosing that side effect to his or her patient. The physician's actions are judged against the actions of his or her peers in the same specialty. Contrary to this perspective, in a growing number of states, informed consent is viewed from the perspective of the patient. If a side effect would be significant to a patient, it should be disclosed to the patient. The fact that other physicians in the same specialty do not disclose a particular side effect or consequence of a drug or medical procedure does not relieve each individual physician of responsibility to communicate information that a patient would consider significant. Under this standard, the physician is required to disclose as much information as necessary to enable the patient to make a knowledgeable decision. This obligation centers on the fundamental right of a patient to make his or her own healthcare decisions based on full knowledge of the facts. In some states, medical disclosure panels have been formed to develop lists of material risks for each type of surgery that must be disclosed for the patient in order to have true informed consent. (See, e.g., Louisiana Medical Disclosure Panel La. R. S. 40: 1299.40.)

Case Discussion

In *Bentley v. Riverside Community Hospital,* the court held that the plaintiffs failed to meet their burden of presenting sufficient evidence to prove that the hospital personnel had a duty to ask the patient whether she was pregnant immediately before the radiologist administered radioiodine therapy to treat symptoms of Graves' disease, or hyperthyroidism. The court concluded that it was the physician's duty to obtain informed consent for the radioiodine therapy and it was not delegable.

Source: Bentley v. Riverside Comm. Hosp., No. E037566 (Cal. App. Dist. 4 07/31/2006).

■ Exceptions to the Duty to Disclose

Before performing most invasive and diagnostic procedures, the patient should give informed consent authorizing the test or procedure. Usually this consent is obtained in writing. However, there may be circumstances where consent is not necessary. There may also be circumstances where there is not time or the opportunity to obtain informed consent. When the decision is made to forgo obtaining informed consent, the healthcare provider must show why consent was not necessary or why it was impossible to obtain from the patient or someone legally authorized to consent on behalf of the patient. Documentation is the best form of defense.

Minor Procedures

When patients are admitted to the hospital, they ordinarily sign an admission form. This form usually contains language authorizing hospital personnel to provide care and treatment to the patient. This avoids the necessity of asking for consent every time a minor procedure is performed. Further, as has already been explained, minor procedures with minimal side effects do not require written informed consent. Procedures in this category include activities such as providing general nursing care and assistance, minor procedures such as drawing blood, and simple diagnostic tests that do not involve great risk (e.g., a chest X-ray).

Emergencies

The most important exception to the informed consent rule pertains to emergency situations. In the case of a medical emergency where the patient is unable to communicate with caregivers, lifesaving treatment ordinarily may be given without the patient's consent. The law implies consent in most emergency circumstances on the theory that if the patient were able or if a qualified legal representative were present, he or she would give consent. If the patient could suffer significant harm if treatment is delayed while family is located, the physician may go forward with treatment. This exception may apply, for example, to the unconscious automobile accident victim who requires emergency surgery. However, this exception does not apply if evidence exists to indicate that the patient (or the patient's legal representative) would refuse the treatment.

If the patient is coherent enough to converse (e.g., through gestures or conversation) or if the patient's family can be located, then the physician should not rely on the emergency treatment exception. Furthermore, if there is evidence that the patient would not wish the particular treatment (e.g., a living will expressing a desire to forego cardiopulmonary resuscitation, or CPR), then the emergency exception likely will not apply. In such situations, hospital administration should get involved to assist in resolving the problem.

Some states provide immunity to a physician who fails to obtain the patient's consent to treatment under certain emergency circumstances. For example, a physician may not be held liable for civil damages for injury or death caused in an emergency situation occurring in a physician's office or in a hospital due to failure to obtain informed consent under conditions such as the following:

1. The patient is unconscious.
2. The physician reasonably believes that the procedure should be undertaken immediately.
3. There was insufficient time to fully inform the patient or to obtain consent from a person authorized to act on behalf of the patient. (Check specific state laws.)

In the case of an emergency, the physician does not sign the consent form on behalf of the patient. Rather, the law implies the patient's consent from the existence of the emergency.

Therapeutic Privilege Exception

A controversial exception to the obligation to disclose all the risks of a proposed treatment may exist when the physician believes that informing the patient of such risks poses such a threat of harm to the patient that disclosure would be unwise or dangerous. This may occur in situations in which the physician fears that the patient will become so ill or emotionally distraught upon learning of the risks that disclosure of the information would be harmful or would interfere with the patient's ability to make a rational decision. The important question for the physician in this circumstance is whether the physician is making a sound medical judgment that the disclosure would pose a risk to the patient's well-being or would interfere with the patient's ability to make a rational decision. This exception flies in the face of the fundamental principle of self-determination, and the courts have never fully endorsed it.

Waiver

Occasionally, patients may prefer to forgo a discussion of the risks of a proposed treatment. Rather, these patients want to simply trust their doctors to do the best for them. In such a circumstance, the patients make a conscious decision to choose ignorance rather than information. Such patients essentially waive their right to informed consent. When the patient clearly chooses not to participate in the consent process, many providers feel comfortable respecting this choice. Courts have agreed with the physicians' decisions in such circumstances. When a patient chooses to waive the right to hear all about the risks of a proposed treatment, the physician is well advised to document such waiver thoroughly in the medical record and to give the patient a number of opportunities to change his or her mind.

■ Documentation

In all cases in which informed consent is obtained, the consent should be well documented in the patient's medical record. The person who obtained the consent, usually the physician, should prepare this documentation. In the case of emergencies, the existence of the emergency and the justification for failing to obtain consent from either the patient or a family member should also be explained.

■ Who May Give Consent?

Competent Patients

A legal and effective informed consent requires that the individual have decision-making capability. The analysis first begins with the question of the competency of the patient. For the purpose of consenting to medical treatment, competency may be defined as the ability to understand the nature and consequences of the procedure or treatment that the patient is being asked to undergo. The general rule is that a person is presumed to be competent unless there is valid reason to believe otherwise. If the patient is competent, then he or she may consent to any and all medical treatment. If the patient is incompetent for any reason, then consent must be obtained elsewhere.

Any number of reasons may cause incompetency. For example, individuals under the legal age of consent (18 years of age) are automatically deemed incompetent to consent to most medical treatment. (Note that this may not apply in states that permit minors the right to consent to medical treatment relating to sexually transmitted diseases and other reproductive health issues such as birth control.) Some states provide that minors who have entered into a valid marriage or who are on active duty in the U.S. armed forces or who have been declared emancipated pursuant to a court decision are competent to make healthcare decisions.

Another example of incompetency is when a court of law determines that a patient lacks the capability to make medical decisions. These individuals usually have a "conservator of the person" appointed for them. State laws vary regarding the appointment and authority of conservators. Before relying upon the consent of a conservator, explore the laws in your own particular state.

Incompetency may also exist in an elderly patient with diminished mental functions, such as a person suffering from senile dementia. A formal court ruling regarding the elderly patient's capability is not usually necessary. If the patient's treating physician or a psychiatrist is able to state that the patient lacks capability, consent may be obtained elsewhere, such as from a surrogate decision maker. However, if there is any dispute regarding the patient's capability, recourse to the courts may be necessary.

Surrogate Decision Maker

If an individual is thought to be incapable (incompetent) to consent to the medical treatment being offered, consent must be obtained in some other fashion. Alternative sources for consent depend on the reason the patient is incompetent. For example, when the patient is incompetent because of age (i.e., the patient is younger than 18), the healthcare provider turns to the parent or legal guardian for consent. If a court has deemed the patient incompetent and a conservator of the person has been appointed, then the healthcare provider looks to the conservator for consent. If the patient is deemed incompetent because of mental incompetency, either temporary (e.g., unconsciousness due to an automobile accident) or permanent (e.g., senility), a hierarchy of individuals who may be capable of consenting exists. In such a circumstance, the healthcare provider should look to the following individuals, known as surrogate decision makers, to make the decision on behalf of the patient. Surrogate decision makers include the following:

1. An adult whom the patient has appointed to make healthcare decisions pursuant to state law (e.g., through a durable power of attorney for health care)

2. A conservator appointed by a court to make medical decisions
3. The nearest relative (e.g., spouse, parent, adult child, siblings, aunts and uncles, cousins).

Other terms commonly used include *healthcare agent, healthcare proxy, healthcare representative,* and *healthcare surrogate.*

When none of these individuals exist, resort to the courts for judicial permission to perform the procedure may be necessary. (It is a misconception that two physicians may agree to the need for particular treatment and consent to it on behalf of the patient when the patient is incompetent and when no surrogate decision maker can be found. Rather, either the emergency consent rule applies or the physicians must obtain a court order authorizing the procedure. In these circumstances, legal counsel should be consulted regarding specific state laws that may apply.)

Evidence of the Patient's Desire

If the patient has made an informed decision regarding treatment before the onset of incompetency, that decision should be given effect even after the patient loses competency. For example, a competent patient who instructs his or her physician to withhold CPR and has a written do-not-resuscitate order (DNR) should have those wishes respected if the patient then loses consciousness and suffers a cardiac arrest.

A living will is a declaration, signed by the patient when competent, stating his or her wishes as to the type and extent of medical treatment he or she wishes to receive. Through this document, a competent adult can provide information and direction to others regarding healthcare treatment in the event that the individual is unable to make decisions. All states have enacted some type of law that permits competent adults to make some type of healthcare decisions in advance, which would take effect at a later date without any involvement of a court or other surrogate decision maker. Unless the living will complies with the standards established by the state in which the patient is located, the living will has no legal binding effect.

Some patients may have signed an advance healthcare directive that includes a living will and a medical durable power of attorney that designates a healthcare proxy, healthcare surrogate, or healthcare representative. A **living will** is a document signed by the competent patient that expresses his or her future healthcare wishes to be carried out when he or she can no longer make such decisions. A **medical durable power of attorney** allows a patient to choose someone to make medical decisions on his or her behalf when the patient is unable to do so. These directives are usually typewritten forms or documents that comply with individual state laws. When an advance directive complies with state law, the physician may be required to follow the wishes of the patient that are expressed within that document. Further, state law may provide healthcare providers with protections from liability when the advance healthcare directive is followed. Providers should carefully check the law in their state to determine the extent to which the advance healthcare directive is binding upon them.

■ Forgoing Life-Sustaining Treatment

When the patient is incapable of making a decision, another person is identified to make the decision on the patient's behalf (i.e., the surrogate decision maker described above). The surrogate decision maker must be motivated solely by an interest in the welfare of the incompetent patient. When the patient has expressed his or her desires, these statements should guide the surrogate decision maker. When a patient has left clear evidence of his or her wishes, the surrogate decision maker should follow these wishes. However, just as the adult competent patient has the right to refuse or to decide not to receive treatment, either because it involves great pain or discomfort or is particularly intrusive or because the patient feels the time has come for treatment to stop altogether, the surrogate decision maker has similar rights.

∎ ∎ ∎ What If?

You are in the room when the physician discusses with the patient the available treatment and the material risks of having the medical procedure recommended for the treatment of cancer. You notice that she fails to discuss treatment that other physicians have used. When the physician leaves, the patient says that she will just take her chances and not have any treatment.
1. What should you do?
2. Ethically do you have an obligation to be a patient advocate?
3. What is the ethical dilemma if you discuss other treatment options with the patient?

Despite the considerable publicity that has surrounded right-to-die issues in recent years, most patients do not leave clear evidence of their wishes. The patient may never have thought about the question or may not have been comfortable discussing his or her feelings with family members. Most courts permit other individuals to consent on the patient's behalf in these circumstances. The first and most famous case to discuss the authority of a surrogate decision maker is the *Quinlan* decision. In that case, the Supreme Court of New Jersey authorized the father of Karen Anne Quinlan to consent to have his irreversibly comatose daughter removed from a respirator. The court permitted this even though the treating physician testified that the patient would die without the respirator and that it was not the custom or practice to remove such patients under those circumstances. Given her poor prognosis, the court found no state interest that could override the patient's right to refuse treatment, which her father was exercising on her behalf. Other courts have since followed the New Jersey ruling and have permitted discontinuance of life support systems for irreversibly comatose patients [5].

When an incompetent patient is severely debilitated but not terminally ill or comatose, courts have been more reluctant to withhold medical care at the direction of the family. A significant case in this area of law is *Cruzan v. Harmon* [6]. On the night of January 11, 1983, Nancy Cruzan lost control of her car as she was driving down a road in Jasper County, Missouri. The car overturned, and Nancy was found lying face down in a ditch without detectable heartbeat or respiration. Paramedics were able to restore her breathing and heart rate at the accident site, and she was transported to a hospital unconscious. She remained in a coma for approximately 3 weeks and then progressed to an unconscious state in which she was able to take some nutrition by mouth. To ease feeding and further the recovery, surgeons implanted a feeding tube directly into her stomach. After it became apparent that Nancy had virtually no chance of regaining her mental faculties, her parents asked the hospital to stop the artificial feedings. The hospital refused to honor this request without court approval. The case made its way through the court system from the trial court level to the Missouri Supreme Court, and then on to the U.S. Supreme Court. The Missouri Supreme Court ruled that in the absence of **clear and convincing evidence** of Nancy's wishes, the state's interest in preserving life outweighed her parents' right to refuse the lifesaving treatment. For that reason, the Missouri Supreme Court refused to permit the removal of the feeding tube. The U.S. Supreme Court, in reviewing the Missouri Supreme Court's decision, supported the analysis of the Missouri court. The U.S. Supreme Court concluded that although the U.S. Constitution supports the right to refuse treatment, that right is not absolute. States may set reasonable limits on the exercise of personal freedoms.

Some states permit surrogate decision makers broad authority to refuse or withdraw life-sustaining measures, including intravenous drips, ventilators, antibiotics, and similar treatments. However, in all circumstances, the comfort of the patient should be considered. Comfort measures, such as pain medications, may not be withheld from a dying patient.

■ Special Circumstances

Federal law specifically addresses the use of restraints in nursing home settings. In a nursing home, special consent is required before the use of most types of restraints. In addition, the Joint Commission on Accreditation of Healthcare Organizations, which accredits many hospitals and other healthcare entities, has very specific requirements regarding the application of and consent to restraints (Box 4-4).

Many states have laws that permit minors, whether emancipated or not, to consent to treatment for sexually transmitted diseases. In addition, many states give minors the authority to consent to birth control and other matters relating to pregnancy. A minor's ability to consent varies from state to state. Some states require parental notification, such as in the case of abortion.

Patients admitted to mental health facilities have special rights regarding consent. A patient may not ordinarily be held and treated against his or her will unless careful attention is paid to complying with state and federal laws regarding involuntary commitment. It is a generally accepted principle of mental health law that even an involuntarily committed patient (i.e., in general, one who has been deemed to present a clear and present danger to oneself or another) retains the limited ability to refuse certain types of medical care, such as electroconvulsive therapy ("shock treatment") and psychosurgeries such as lobotomies. State law determines the extent of these rights.

Box 4-4 | Special Circumstances Relating to Consent

- Restraints
- Reproductive rights
- Mental health treatment
- Research studies
- Law enforcement

Federal law prohibits the performance of any sort of experimental treatment for purposes of research without the express written consent of the patient or the patient's surrogate decision maker. Further, the consent form that is used in such circumstances must comply with all the disclosure requirements set forth in federal law. These disclosure requirements are extensive, which accounts for the lengthy and detailed consent forms used in research studies.

It is not uncommon that police officers bring a prisoner or suspect to a healthcare facility requesting that a particular medical procedure be performed on the individual. For example, a request may be made to withdraw blood for drug tests or to pump the patient's stomach for collection of evidence in a drug search. Such invasive procedures may violate the patient's **Fifth Amendment** right against self-incrimination and the **Sixth Amendment** rights against unreasonable searches and seizures by law enforcement. Furthermore, if the patient objects, physical force or restraints may be necessary to enable the procedure to be performed. This may result in injury to the patient. Before using such force or restraint or going against the patient's wishes, the healthcare provider should check hospital or laboratory policy and state laws to determine how best to proceed.

How Consent Should Be Obtained

The obligation to provide the information necessary for the patient to give informed consent is the responsibility of the patient's physician. Other healthcare employees involved in the consent process should merely serve as witnesses to the patient's signing of the consent form and can document discussions of informed consent.

If the patient does not speak English, every effort must be made to provide an interpreter, either in person or by telephone. (The patient is not able to give informed consent if he or she does not understand what is being said.) The institution in which the patient is receiving treatment should have a policy to address use of and access to interpreters.

When the individual giving consent is unable to sign the consent form (e.g., if a spouse provides consent over the telephone), the conversation with the surrogate decision maker should be well documented in the patient's medical record. Some facilities require that two witnesses hear the telephone consent and that documentation describing the discussion with the decision be made a part of the chart. An explanation should be given as to why the patient or surrogate decision maker is unable to sign the consent form. Furthermore, it is a wise practice to document all stages of the informed consent process in the medical record. Documentation of a patient's informed consent is essential for the protection of the healthcare provider and the institution.

■ Conclusion

Let us revisit the case scenario in light of the information provided in this chapter. We know that, ordinarily, an adult patient is presumed competent unless we have reason to believe otherwise. We also know to look for a formal document, such as a durable power of attorney for health care or a conservatorship of the person, which may give another person the authority to make medical decisions when the patient is incompetent. If such a document does not exist, a family member can make decisions on behalf of an incompetent patient. Many states have laws designating the order of who can give consent. We also know that obtaining informed consent is the physician's responsibility and that other healthcare providers can act as witnesses to the signing of the consent form.

Let us apply these lessons to the facts of the opening scenario. We see that Mrs. Richards has advanced Alzheimer's disease, which raises doubts as to whether she has the capability to consent to the colonoscopy. The physician should evaluate the patient's ability to understand the risks and benefits of the procedure. If she cannot understand them, the physician would conclude that the patient does not have the capability to consent. The husband should then be asked about the existence of a durable power of attorney for health care or a court-appointed conservatorship of the person. If none of these exists, the husband may be asked to sign the consent form.

When Mr. Richards began asking Susan questions about the procedure, Susan recognized that Mr. Richards did not appear to have a good understanding of the risks and benefits. Perhaps he never had the chance to speak to a physician about it, or perhaps he didn't understand the explanation given to him by the doctor. At this point, Susan should not attempt to explain the medical aspects of the procedure. Instead, she should tell Mr. Richards that it would be better if a doctor answered his questions. Susan should then find the radiologist and request that he speak directly to Mr. Richards to answer his questions. After the radiologist speaks to him, Susan may then observe Mr. Richards sign the consent form and then sign her own name as the witness.

As we can see from this scenario, knowledge of the principles of informed consent is essential to achieving the goal of providing patients with high-quality medical care. Patients deserve to have their questions answered before submitting to any medical procedure. Patients also deserve to be given enough information to make an informed decision about whether to agree to the procedure. Even though the healthcare worker may not agree with the choices made by the patient, the law requires that the worker respect these choices. Failure to meet informed consent obligations may result in significant liability to the healthcare provider and the employer.

■ ■ ■ Pertinent Points

1. The competent adult patient has the right to accept or refuse medical procedures that the physician recommends to him or her. This right may be restricted only in limited circumstances.
2. The duty to obtain the patient's informed consent rests with the individual performing the procedure such as the physician, nurse practitioner, or physician's assistant.
3. When the patient lacks the capability to consent to medical treatment, consent ordinarily can be obtained from a surrogate decision maker. If living will or natural death legislation has been enacted in your state, then you should ask the patient or family members whether the patient has signed a document addressing the patient's wishes regarding medical treatment.
4. In 1914, Judge Cardozo made the famous statement, "Every human being of adult years and sound mind has the right to determine what shall be done with his own body."
5. A battery occurs whenever a person intentionally touches another without permission.
6. The informed consent disclosure requirements include the following:
   a. Name and proposed treatment
   b. Material risks and consequences
   c. Alternatives
   d. Consequences of refusal of treatment.
7. Exceptions to informed consent include emergencies, minor procedures, waiver, and the therapeutic privilege exception.
8. A living will is a document signed by a competent patient that expresses the person's future healthcare wishes to be carried out when he or she can no longer make such decisions.
9. A medical durable power of attorney or healthcare proxy allows a patient to choose someone to make medical decisions on his or her behalf when the patient is unable to do so.

10. The physician performing the surgery or procedure should obtain informed consent from the patient.
11. A DNR order may be a part of the living will and must have a physician's order that should be periodically updated.

▪ ▪ ▪ Study Questions

1. Define battery and give an example.
2. Discuss the foundation for the informed consent doctrine.
3. Outline the informed consent requirements. Obtain a facility's consent form and discuss the various requirements.
4. What is the responsibility of the allied health professional with regard to informed consent forms and the process of obtaining informed consent?
5. Discuss the term *implied consent* and give an example.
6. Define the terms *competency* and *incompetency*. Discuss the general rule related to competency.
7. What is a surrogate decision maker? Who can be a surrogate decision maker?
8. Discuss two important legal cases relating to life-sustaining treatment and their impact on the healthcare arena. Present these cases to the class.
9. What is an advance directive? Obtain a copy of a living will and medical durable power of attorney or healthcare proxy used in a local healthcare facility and present them to the class.
10. Define the special circumstances related to consent and how they affect patient care.
11. Research on the Internet and find your state law on advance directives.
12. Research and discuss a case you found based on a lack of informed consent.

▪ ▪ ▪ References

1. Schloendorff v. Soc'y of N.Y. Hosp., 105 N.E. 92 (N.Y. 1914).
2. Cobbs v. Grant, 502 P.2d 1 (Cal. 1972).
3. Canterbury v. Spence, 464 F.2d 772 (D.C. Cir. 1972).
4. Truman v. Thomas, 27 Cal.3d 285 (1980).
5. *In re* Quinlan, 355 A.2d 647 (N.J. 1976).
6. Cruzan v. Harmon, 76 S.W.2d 408 (Mo. 1988), *aff'd,* Cruzan v. Dir., Mo. Dept. of Health, 497 U.S. 261 (1990).

■ ■ ■ **Resources**

Aiken, Tonia D. *Legal, Ethical, and Political Issues in Nursing*, Chap. 11,
    Informed Consent (2nd ed.). Philadelphia: F. A. Davis Company.
Compassion & Choices Hemlock Society, www.compassionandchoices.org.
U.S. Living Will Registry, www.uslivingwillregistry.com.

5

Documentation and the Allied Health Professional

Key Chapter Concepts

■
■
■

Flow Sheets
Focus Charting
Graphic Sheet
Health Insurance Portability and Accountability Act (HIPAA)
Intake and Output Sheet
Integrated Progress Notes
Kardex
Medical Records
PIE Charting
Plan of Care/Nursing Care Plan
Progress Notes
SOAP/SOAPIE

Objectives

At the conclusion of this chapter, the reader will be able to:

■
■
■

1. Define purposes of the medical record.
2. Discuss major uses of the medical record.
3. Outline commonly used documentation forms, including a nursing care plan and Kardex.
4. Define common guidelines for charting.
5. Discuss legal implications of releasing confidential information about the patient.
6. Discuss the advantages and disadvantages of electronic charting.

■ Why Do We Have Medical Records?

The medical record of a patient contains a large amount of personal and medical information. The information is collected in a medical record for many reasons, including the following:
- To help the doctors reach a diagnosis of the patient's medical or psychological condition
- To enable the nurses, therapists, and other healthcare providers to develop a list of the patient's problems
- To provide a place to record observations about the patient
- To record information about the treatments and care provided to the patient
- To record responses or reactions of the patient to care.

Medical records are usually created wherever a patient receives care from a healthcare professional. These locations include medical centers, hospitals, homes, nursing homes, doctors' offices, outpatient clinics, urgent care centers, therapy centers (e.g., physical, developmental, and occupational therapy), and crisis intervention centers. The principles of recording information in a chart are similar in all these locations.

The medical record's primary purpose is to provide a format for healthcare providers to communicate with one another about the patient. Such healthcare providers may include dental hygienists, X-ray technicians, ultrasound technicians, nurses, doctors, dietitians, therapists, aides, social workers, and assistants. The chart allows healthcare providers who are seeing the patient at different times to learn what others have done for the patient. For example, the nurse's notes, nursing assistant's recordings, and flow sheets give the physician information about the patient's status that will affect the orders that the physician writes. A home health aide can use the entries of a physical therapist who visits a patient at home to reinforce the exercises that have been taught to the patient.

Case Scenario

A Florida woman died in a nursing home after having been a patient for five years. She was 94 years old at the time of admission. During her stay, she was totally dependent on skilled nursing and catheter care, but the level of care was apparently very poor. Record keeping was severely deficient, sometimes with gaps of weeks between the required daily nursing notes. Existing notes were often internally conflicting or in conflict with other pieces of the decedent's chart that other caretakers had recorded on the same day. The woman suffered a broken ankle, broken hip, torn rotator cuff, numerous stage IV bedsores (the most serious type), and severe contractures while in the home. She died of congestive heart failure, with sepsis (blood infection) listed as a secondary cause of death. The parties settled for $800,000 two days before trial [1]. Frequency of charting was an issue in this case, which we will discuss in more detail later in the chapter.

■ Purposes of Documentation

The information recorded in the medical record is used to do the following:
1. Identify the patient's problems and strengths
2. Plan care for the patient
3. Record care that is given to the patient
4. Fulfill legal obligations to record pertinent information about the patient

   Documentation is used to do the following:
1. Provide evidence of the provision of quality nursing care
2. Provide evidence of the nurse's legal responsibilities to the patient
3. Record information for personal health protection
4. Provide evidence of standards, rules, regulations, and laws regarding nursing, medical, and allied health practices
5. Record statistical information for standards and research
6. Provide cost-benefit reduction information
7. Provide risk management information
8. Provide information for student learning experiences
9. Provide evidence of protection of patient rights
10. Record professional and ethical conduct and responsibility
11. Provide data to determine the type of care needed on discharge
12. Provide data for planning future health care
13. Provide data on nursing and medical history for future admissions
14. Provide data for quality-of-care review
15. Provide data for continuing education and research
16. Provide data for billing and reimbursement
17. Provide data to record nursing care, which forms the basis of evaluation by the Joint Commission on Accreditation for Healthcare Organizations (JCAHO) and other federal or state agencies
18. Provide communication between the responsible nursing professionals and other practitioners contributing to managing patient care (Box 5-1)

Box 5-1 | Routine Records Found in a Patient's Chart

1. Admission sheet
2. Emergency room record
3. History and physical
4. Discharge summary
5. Consultations
6. Operative report
7. Laboratory results
8. X-ray reports
9. Diagnostic study reports (e.g., CT scan, MRI, ultrasound)
10. Nurses' notes
11. Physician orders
12. Progress notes
13. Vital sign sheet, graphic records
14. Intake and output sheet
15. Medication administration record
16. Pathology reports
17. Autopsy report
18. Respiratory therapists' notes
19. Physical and occupational therapists' notes
20. Observation sheet
21. Flow sheets
22. Physician's office records
23. Ambulance run sheet (may not be in the records unless ambulances are part of facility's services)
24. Kardex
25. Plan of care

Patient Problem Identification

The patient's chart consists of information about the patient's problems, which may include physical and emotional changes that affect health status. Strengths may be defined as the areas of health or the patient's abilities to care for self. For example, a patient in a nursing home may be able to wash her face and hands but may require assistance washing her back and legs. The information recorded by the nursing assistants enables others to identify the patient's abilities and needs.

Plan Patient Care

Once the patient's problems and strengths are identified, the staff involved in the patient's care are then able to plan the care. The plan of care can be documented in several different formats.

A commonly used format is a nursing care plan and critical pathway, which are described in more detail below. Also, the discharge summary states a plan of care after the patient is discharged from a facility for physician's services and other healthcare, psychological, or social services.

Record of Care Provided

The medical record provides a format for recording care provided to the patient. The dental hygienist records the care associated with cleaning the teeth. The home health aide documents the assistance provided in dressing and grooming. The medical assistant documents the patient's initial complaints on arrival at the doctor's or nurse practitioner's office. The healthcare providers use the medical record to prove that care is given that is important for reimbursement purposes and to show that the standard of care is being followed.

Legal Document

The medical record (or medical chart) is a legal document and is used to determine whether healthcare providers carried out their obligations to the patient and followed policies, procedures, guidelines, and standards. It must not be thrown out, altered, or destroyed. The actual pieces of paper belong to the healthcare facility that provides the care to the patient. The patient owns the information that is recorded in the chart.

If the patient wants to read his or her record, tell the nurse, who may want to discuss this with the physician before showing the patient the records. Also, check to see whether your hospital has a policy and procedure on allowing patients to see their charts while in the hospital. After the patient has been discharged from the facility, the patient may obtain a copy of the medical record by requesting a copy. The facility may charge a fee for duplication.

■ Components of the Medical Record

Plan of Care

When the patient is admitted to the facility, an initial assessment is performed. The data collected are used to identify the patient's problems and to plan the care. The plan of care may be recorded in a hospital or nursing home in the form of a nursing care plan (Case Example 5-1). The care plan usually defines the following:

1. The patient's problems
2. The outcomes or goals to be achieved
3. The interventions or steps to be carried out to achieve the outcomes

Case Example 5-1

When Mary Quigley is admitted to the nursing home, she is unsteady on her feet and at risk of falling. The nursing care plan identified for her is as follows:

Problem: High risk for falls on the basis of a fall risk assessment.

Outcome: Will not fall during her stay at the facility.

Interventions:
1. Determine the reason for wanting to wander or get out of bed, such as need to use bathroom, pain, high energy level or anxiety.
2. Identify the patient as fall prone by labeling the bed, the wristband, and the medical record.
3. Place recognizable symbols on the patient's door to direct the patient back to his or her own room.
4. Use bed-exit alarms.
5. Place the mattress on floor.
6. Keep the call bell accessible.
7. Remind the patient and family to call for assistance to get out of bed.

The nursing care plan identifies the high priority problems that are pertinent to the patient's condition. The nursing care plan changes over time as the patient's needs change. After the registered nurse establishes the care plan, the licensed practical nurse may add additional information.

Kardex

The care plan may be combined on the same document with a Kardex. The Kardex is an abbreviated listing of the care elements specific to the patient. The Kardex commonly defines the following:

1. The type of diet
2. The patient's activity level
3. The amount of assistance the patient needs for bathing
4. The treatments to be performed

Dugan, White, and Cusick [2] reported on nursing assistants' use of a Kardex to identify the following:

1. The special equipment used by the resident
2. The need for a wheelchair
3. The application schedule for splints, cones, or other rehabilitation devices

4. Other assistive devices needed by the resident
5. The level of assistance the resident needs for activities of daily living

The Kardex provides a level of consistency in assignments in facilities and reduces the potential errors of floating nursing assistants. The Kardex is changed as the needs of the patient change.

Progress Notes

The format and design of progress notes have gone through enormous changes in the past decade. For many years, entries into medical records were written in a **narrative format.** In other words, entries were written as paragraphs with no particular organization, other than by date of entry. As health care became more complex and the need to transmit more and more information occurred, the narrative note came under attack. The criticisms of the narrative note have focused primarily on its unstructured format. It can be very difficult to locate information about a specific subject in a long narrative note. The documentation of narrative notes is very time consuming. Also, sometimes too much or too little information is documented.

SOAP Format

In the 1960s, the physician Lawrence Weed created a system of organizing entries in outpatient charts: the SOAP format. This system consists of a problem list and progress notes. The problem list is an ongoing listing of the patient's current and resolved problems. The progress note is broken down into four components:
S: Subjective (what the patient says)
O: Objective (what the healthcare provider observes)
A: Assessment (the conclusion of the healthcare provider about the label for the problem)
P: Plan (what will be done about the problem).

A nurse working in a facility that uses SOAP charting may make the following entry:
S: "I have pain in my abdomen"
O: Rubbing abdomen, grimacing
A: Abdominal pain
P: Give pain medication

The SOAP system usually includes the concept of integrated progress notes. These are notes that several types of healthcare providers—such as nurses, doctors, physical therapists, dietitians, and others—write.

In the early 1980s, the limitations of the SOAP system became apparent as the components of the SOAP note were studied. The basic SOAP note does not include a way to document the interventions carried out to address the problem, nor does it include a framework for documenting the patient's response. Therefore, the SOAP system has been modified to include the following:

I: Intervention (what was done about the problem)

E: Evaluation (the patient's reaction)

The full SOAPIE note may look like this:

S: "I have pain in my abdomen"

O: Rubbing abdomen, grimacing

A: Abdominal pain

P: Give pain medication

I: Demerol 75 mg IM given

E: States she felt better an hour after receiving injection

While the new SOAPIE note provides a full framework for documenting information about the patient, the sheer length of the note makes it cumbersome to use (Box 5-2).

Box 5-2 | Tips for Documentation

1. Chart the care you give.
2. Chart the facts; use concrete and specific information.
3. Quote patient's own words: "My stomach hurts."
4. Do not make assumptions.
5. Use ink.
6. Do not chart for anyone else.
7. Use approved facility abbreviations.
8. Know the facility's policies and procedures on documentation.
9. Document calls to other healthcare providers and the content of your message.
10. Chart late entries according to facility policy.
11. Do not falsify records.
12. Do not write on the chart, "Incident report written in patient's records."
13. Use intercommunication sheets or incident/occurrence variance reports for issues relating to risk management or legal issues to protect the confidentiality of the information.
14. Initial and sign each entry.
15. Record information that shows the patient is noncompliant or uncooperative.
16. "If it wasn't charted, it wasn't done" (the judge and jury commonly make this assumption).
17. Confidentiality is a primary concern.

PIE Charting

As the limitations of SOAPIE became clear and the time associated with writing either lengthy narrative notes or detailed SOAPIE notes became apparent, different charting systems emerged. Two of them, **PIE** and **focus charting,** are in common use.

PIE charting structures the progress note into *P* for problem, *I* for intervention, and *E* for evaluation. For example:
P: Abdominal pain
 I: Demerol 75 mg IM given
 E: Obtained relief within an hour

Focus Charting

Focus charting uses a column format for the focus, or problem. The note is then organized into *D* for data, *A* for action, and *R* for response. For example:
Focus: Abdominal pain
D: Stating she has pain, clutching abdomen, grimacing
A: Demerol 75 mg IM given
R: States she received relief from pain within an hour

Flow Sheets

As changes were made in the format of the progress note, increasing numbers of flow sheets were developed and put into use in various facilities. A flow sheet is basically a table that consists of information in columns. A common format is to have the time of day running across the top of the page and the data elements or activities running down the length of a page.

Flow sheets on nursing units in hospitals, nursing homes, or home care address many different types of activities and needs. Commonly used flow sheets in hospitals include patient care flow sheets, care provided to a patient in restraints, neurological assessment, and vital signs. In long-term care, flow sheets typically include patient care, vital signs, and weight.

Nursing assistants in hospitals and nursing homes as well as home health aids frequently write on patient care flow sheets. The purpose of the flow sheet is to provide a place in the chart to document the routine aspects of care, including the type of bath given, the patient's activity (bed rest, out of bed, bathroom privileges), and the consumption of food at each meal (type of diet and percentage of food eaten).

Brief entries are written in each column. The form may include codes for entries using brief words or letters such as *C* for complete bath. In contrast, the people entering information on the form may record only their initials, depending on how the form is designed. There is usually a place at the bottom of the form for providers to sign to indicate their initials and full name. This form may be different if adapted for use with a computer.

Graphic Records

A form commonly used by nursing assistants is the **graphic sheet.** In most acute care facilities, the graphic sheet is designed so that several days of data are on one form. The chart is set up so that the time (dates and hours of entries) is across the top of the page, and the vital sign values are in the left column. The form includes an area to document temperature, pulse, respiration, and blood pressure (Table 5-1). In long-term care and home care, the vital signs are taken less often. In these settings, the vital signs are usually written in longhand, not graphed, unless computerized charting is used.

■ Intake and Output

Hospitals commonly use forms to keep track of intake and output. The forms often include an area for the nurse to record the intake from intravenous fluid solutions and intravenous medications, such as antibiotics diluted in minibags. The nursing assistant may be involved in documenting the amount of fluids that the patient drank or the drainage from tubes. It is important that this information is as accurate as possible. A discrepancy between the patient's intake and output may result in the administration of medications or fluids to try to reestablish a balance.

■ Guidelines for Charting

A few good commonsense rules govern the entry of information into the medical record.

Table 5-1 | Example of a Graphic Sheet

Date	Temperature	Pulse	Respirations	Blood Pressure
12/3	98.7	84	20	120/86
12/10	99.0	88	22	130/90

Chart the Care You Give

In each type of patient care area, there are different rules about the frequency of charting and the types of information that should be recorded in the medical record. While charting every shift is standard in hospitals, charting certain information every day or every week may be acceptable in long-term care. Although nurses' notes are not commonly written every day in long-term care, the nursing assistants often use the patient care flow sheet daily.

In the case scenario at the beginning of this chapter, the absence of the required documentation complicated the defense of the nursing home. The large settlement for a patient who was 90 years of age may have been the result of the inability to point to the medical record to assert that the patient had received appropriate care.

Do Not Falsify, Tamper With, or Alter Records

The medical record should be an accurate document that truthfully records the care provided. Falsifying the medical record can result in serious consequences to the patient and, for the healthcare providers, in a lawsuit, as Case Example 5-2 illustrates. Also, disciplinary actions may result from falsification of documents. Healthcare providers must also depend on the information supplied to them as being truthful and, unless they find it to be false, accept it as is, as demonstrated in the Poe case [3]. In Poe, plaintiff alleged that physicians and staff falsified his medical records by relying on hearsay statements made by his girlfriend and sister when his medical history was taken in 2001 and 2002. Plaintiff complaint was dismissed.

In the Poe case, the plaintiff alleged that the doctors and medical staff from the hospital falsified his medical records by relying on hearsay statements from the plaintiff's sister and girlfriend when they filled out his medical history on two separate occasions. Plaintiff was upset about references in the medical record stating that he threatened to harm himself and others, that he had a history of violence, and that he was depressed and suicidal. There is no allegation that the medical personnel knew the information given to them was false. The plaintiff was not in custody at the time but was at the time of the filing of the claim. The plaintiff sued under 42 U.S.C. §1983, which addresses a deprivation of a right secured by the U.S. Constitution by a person acting under color of state law. The hospital staff were not state actors and worked in a private hospital and cannot be used under

42 U.S.C. §1983. The court dismissed the case. The court also dismissed the case because it failed to state a claim for relief and the allegations were frivolous.

Case Example 5-2

The patient was admitted to the defendant hospital's behavioral science unit one day after slitting his wrist in an attempted suicide. The patient continued having suicidal thoughts while in the defendant hospital. Four days after admission, the patient took a plastic garbage can liner that was in the room and suffocated himself. The hospital's employees performed as many as 12 bed checks while the patient lay dead in his bed. The patient's death was only discovered when the hospital's staff attempted to awaken him the following morning. The Pennsylvania jury found that the hospital and the defendant physician, who treated the patient a decade earlier for depression, were grossly negligent in treating the decedent. The plaintiff received $800,000 in compensatory damages from both defendants and $800,000 in punitive damages against the hospital [4]. (Punitive damages are designed to punish the healthcare provider for conduct that is considered to be grossly negligent. Insurance policies usually do not provide coverage for punitive damages, so these awards are paid out of the pocket of the defendant.)

▪▪▪ What If?

A. You see a coworker who is your friend swapping her notes and rewriting them.
B. You know the nursing assistant did not take vital signs but has fabricated them and is documenting these false vital signs on patients' charts.
C. You see a nurse documenting a late entry two days after a patient died.
   1. What should you do in each scenario?
   2. What is the ethical dilemma in each scenario?
   3. Are there potential legal issues that can arise? What are they?

Use Ink

Because the chart is a legal document, entries must be permanent. Pencil entries are not acceptable.

Corrections

If incorrect information is accidentally entered, the format in many facilities for correcting the mistake is to draw a line through the entry and then write the date and the person's initials above the entry.

Avoid words that indicate negligence, such as *error, mistaken entry, miscalculated, intentionally,* or *by accident.*

The original entry should still be readable. The use of heavy black marker or correction fluid is not an acceptable method of changing the original entry. These correction methods present the appearance of an attempt to cover up or hide an error that affected the patient.

Initial or Sign the Entry

The person who put the information into the medical record should sign the entry. The signing of the entry provides a method of demonstrating accountability for the data and allows someone else to go back to that person to clarify the data.

Record Information with Care

The medical record acts to protect healthcare providers when a patient has a bad outcome from care. The legal system includes the premise that the patient should make reasonable efforts to cooperate with healthcare providers and to follow instructions for self care. It is important to document when the patient refuses care.

In dentists' and physicians' offices and other clinics, it is common practice to record missed appointments on a patient's chart. In Case Examples 5-3 and 5-4, the patient's failure to keep appointments and follow instructions was a factor in the successful defense of the lawsuit. Careful recording of missed appointments is essential. This is commonly written as "no show," "DNKA" (did not keep appointment), or "DNS" (did not show). Attempts to reach the patient to reschedule care, including the use of letters, postcards, or phone calls, should be documented in the medical record.

Case Example 5-3

A 60-year-old Georgia truck driver had a wisdom tooth extracted by the defendant dentist. Several weeks later, another dentist diagnosed osteomyelitis (bone infection) and pathological fracture (fracture from a weakened bone) of the patient's lower jaw secondary to a postoperative infection. Surgery had to be performed to remove decayed tissue and bone and to wire the jaw. Other treatment required included intravenous antibiotics, hyperbaric oxygen treatments, and bone grafting to the jaw.

The plaintiff claimed that the extraction was unnecessary and that the defendant failed to give him appropriate postextraction instructions and to diagnose the infection during postoperative visits. The defendant contended that the extraction was necessary, that the plaintiff did not take the antibiotics as instructed, and that he did

Continued

Case Example 5-3—cont'd

not keep all follow-up appointments. The verdict was for the defense [5]. In this case, the specific recording of missed appointments by the office staff of the dentist was a key factor in defending the dentist.

Case Example 5-4

A woman in her early thirties alleged that her dentist was negligent in failing to diagnose and treat periodontal disease and in failing to perform pocket depth probing or take X-rays. The defendant contended that the plaintiff declined X-rays due to the cost and that she did refer the plaintiff to a periodontist. The dentist added to her defense by maintaining that the plaintiff was contributorily negligent in missing dental appointments and that any delay in diagnosis did not affect outcome. The jury returned a defense verdict [6].

Record Unusual Incidents or Events

Unusual events are considered incidents. Descriptions of incidents are critical to document the unusual circumstances in which patients may or may not get hurt. The description of the incident is often used at the time of a lawsuit to determine whether the actions of the healthcare providers were appropriate. The absence of a description of an incident may also be used to assert that a particular event did not occur (Case Examples 5-5 and 5-6).

Case Example 5-5

A 60-year-old retired woman underwent a stress echocardiogram, which included a treadmill test. A week after the treadmill test, which was done in the cardiologist's office, the woman's husband called the doctor to report that she had seriously injured her back when she fell off the treadmill during the test. Neither the cardiologist nor the two technicians present in the room during the test remembered a fall or any other unusual incident occurring at the time. The plaintiff claimed that the technician had negligently instructed her to get off the treadmill while the belt was moving backward, causing her to fall and to suffer a herniated disk. The defendants contended that the plaintiff injured her back sometime after the test and denied that the incident reported by the plaintiff ever happened. The verdict was for the defense [7].

The defense of the cardiologist and the technicians was based on the premise that the lack of documentation of the alleged fall indicated that it did not occur. An injury of this nature would have been recorded in the cardiologist's office notes. Additional statements by the technicians would have also been appropriate.

In another case, the jury in a claim involving a radiology technician returned a defense verdict. The plaintiff was a man in his late sixties who had a stroke affecting his left side. He claimed that the day after his admission, a radiology technician came in to take him to the radiology department for a test. The plaintiff claimed that the technician reached over and grabbed his flaccid left arm to get him onto the stretcher, resulting in a torn rotator cuff of the left shoulder. The plaintiff's family, who were in the room at the time, claimed that they complained to the attending nurse, head nurse, and head physician, none of whom had any recollection of the complaint. There was no documentation of a complaint. The defendant denied the incident happened. The defendant also disputed that the event occurred because the rotator cuff tear was not diagnosed until one year later [8].

■ Incident, Variance, or Occurrence Report

Documentation of incidents typically contains an objective description of the events. The report should be devoid of blame and accusations. For example, the report should not contain statements such as, "This injury occurred because we did not have enough staff to care for the patients," or, "The lab was late as usual on the stat blood work." The incident should be described as soon as possible after the event so that the information is accurate. Serious incidents involving patient injury should be reported up the chain of command. Take care in filing results of diagnostic studies. It is imperative that the results of diagnostic tests are promptly conveyed to the healthcare providers. Delayed reporting of critical results can have a profound impact on the health of a patient (Case Example 5-7).

A Texas jury awarded $67.5 million to a child who lost her left leg after her magnetic resonance imaging (MRI) result was misplaced for more than a day. After a burro attacked her, she underwent surgery to remove part of her intestine. A blood clot had formed on her aorta, cutting off circulation to her leg. The plaintiffs argued that if the results of the MRI test had not been lost for more than a day, the clot could have been detected and the leg saved [9].

　　The accurate filing of reports is an essential responsibility of all staff who handle medical records. Attention to detail, ensuring that the results are not placed on the wrong person's chart, and properly handling the report are important in managing medical records (Case Example 5-8).

Case Example 5-8

In a Pennsylvania case, a 48-year-old woman underwent a mammogram in her gynecologist's office under the direction of Spectrascan employees. A Spectrascan employee misdirected the mammogram report to a pile for routine screening tests rather than the pile for diagnostic tests. The plaintiff claimed that her breast cancer was not diagnosed between February 1995 and October 1995, allowing the cancer to spread to her bones, lungs, and brain. She was not expected to survive. A $33.1 million verdict was reached, with the gynecologist and his practice found 17% at fault and Spectrascan found 83% at fault. The verdict included about $1.1 million in past and future medical expenses and lost wages and $27 million to the plaintiff for pain and suffering. Her husband was awarded $5 million for loss of consortium [10].

■ Confidentiality of the Medical Record

HIPAA

In 1996, Congress enacted HIPAA, which allows for the portability of group insurance coverage. HIPPA allows a person with a preexisting condition who has had continuous health coverage for more than 12 months to leave a job and prevents him or her from being declined for coverage at a new job. Also, HIPAA includes a privacy rule that created national standards to protect patients' and clients' personal health information.

Confidentiality of information is a primary concern of the public. Release of private health information has ruined careers and resulted in public ridicule, social rejection, and economic devastation of individuals and their families. Healthcare professionals have adopted ethical codes that address their responsibility to protect the privacy of patients [11]. However, there are many groups of healthcare providers who do not have formally adopted codes of ethics to guide them in making decisions about revealing patient information. Facility policies and procedures on confidentiality must also be followed. All people involved with patient specific healthcare information are bound by an ethical code, which emphasizes privacy and confidentiality of information [12].

Electronic Charting: Computerized Documentation

The issue of confidentiality assumes new importance as computerization of healthcare information becomes widespread. Security strategies are commonly used to protect information contained in computer systems. Several types of systems are used to restrict access to the computer. The use of cards to activate the terminal or passwords is commonplace. Secondary confidentiality techniques involving biometrics are also being designed. Confidentiality techniques involving retinal (eye) patterns, fingerprints, and circulatory system checks are being developed. Once the user is admitted into the system, the information that can be accessed can be clearly defined. For example, a nursing assistant may be allowed to enter vital sign data but cannot access telephone orders from a physician or read laboratory results.

Potential Legal Problems

Computerized patient records increase the potential for legal problems through the following:
1. Accidental or intentional disclosure of private data to unauthorized individuals
2. Modification or destruction of patient records
3. Entering inaccurate information into the computer
4. Making clinical decisions on the basis of inaccurate information [13]
    Many people believe that the advantages (Box 5-3) of computerizing information outweigh the disadvantages (Box 5-4) and risk to confidentiality, provided that the users carefully respect the patient's rights.

Box 5-3 | **Advantages of Electronic Charting**

The advantages that computerizing patient information provide include the following:
1. Legible entries
2. Instantly accessible records
3. The potential for streamlined documentation
4. The ability to sort and organize the data to show trends in the patient's condition
5. Improved productivity through decreased paperwork time and redundant charting
6. Reduction in record tampering
7. Graphical display of data so that they can be analyzed
8. Support of the use of nursing process and individualization of patient assessment; software can suggest nursing diagnosis on the basis of findings
9. Automatically printed reports
10. Documentation according to standards of care and policies and procedures
11. Availability of data for research projects
12. Allows basing charges on care that is delivered
13. Simultaneous use of patient's records

Box 5-4 | Disadvantages of Electronic Charting

1. Computer downtime due to sudden unexpected failure or routine servicing
2. Size of record (may be voluminous)
3. Acceptance of computerized information when it may be incorrect
4. Confidentiality and security issues
5. Inadequate number of terminals
6. Staff's difficulty in giving up worksheets
7. Costs (e.g., hardware, software, education, licensing fees)

■ Conclusion

The medical record is a rich source of information about the patient. It is a convenient tool for communicating to other healthcare providers the essential information that will help guide their care of the patient. Trends in charting include streamlined progress notes, use of computers, and increased awareness of confidentiality issues.

▪ ▪ ▪ Pertinent Points

1. A primary purpose of the medical record is to provide a format for communication about the needs of the patient.
2. The information in a chart is used to identify the patient's problems and strengths, to plan and record the patient's care, and to fulfill legal obligations to record pertinent information.
3. The nursing care plan identifies the patient's problems, the goals of care, and the steps to be taken to resolve the problems.
4. The Kardex contains a quick reference to identify the needs of the patient and the treatments that have been ordered.
5. Progress notes can be structured in several different ways, including narrative, SOAP, SOAPIE, and PIE.
6. Flow sheets contain tables that are used to record information over time.
7. Forms that may be kept at the patient's bedside include graphic records and intake and output records.
8. Computerized medical records have advantages in that the information is legible, accessible, and streamlined.
9. Disadvantages of computerized medical records relate to confidentiality issues and the risk of destruction of records or entering inaccurate information into the computer.
10. HIPAA created national standards to protect parents' and clients' personal health information.

1. Your friend comments about a mutual acquaintance, "I think Serena had an abortion last week. Since you work as a technician in the OR, have you seen her name on the operating room schedule for an abortion?" How would you respond?
2. Your husband says to you, "Are any of the patients on your unit HIV positive and, if so, who are they?" What do you say?
3. Dietary aides say to you, "You work on Five West. I saw football star Paul Harmon's name as being on your unit. Why is he in the hospital?" How do you answer?
4. When you enter the X-ray waiting area to bring Mr. Watson back to his room, you find him reading his medical record. What do you do?
5. Your supervisor reviews your flow sheet after a patient has fallen out of bed and says, "I want you to chart that the side rails were up before the fall." You know that the rails were down. How do you respond?
6. You observe the unit secretary using correction fluid to change the way she transcribed a medication order. What do you do?
7. Find a healthcare provider who is using the computer for documentation. Ask that person for his or her opinion about the pros and cons of the system. What are its benefits? What are its drawbacks?
8. Use the internet or local law library and ask to see a publication that reports malpractice verdicts. Bring a case involving documentation to class to discuss.
9. Discuss the common types of "incidents" reported in incident, variance, or occurrence reports in your facility.
10. Obtain a copy of your facility's policies and procedures on documentation and discuss them with staff.
11. Discuss how documentation can be improved on your unit or at your facility. Make recommendations to administration.
12. Discuss how documentation problems can be effectively handled at your facility.

▪ ▪ ▪ **References**

1. Laska, L. (Ed.) (1996, January). Elderly woman dies in nursing home. *Medical Malpractice Verdicts, Settlements and Experts*, 26–27.
2. Dugan, M., White, D., & Cusick, P. (1995, April). Care-planning in long-term care. *Nursing Management, 26*(4), 48.
3. Poe v. Nort, No. 1:06CV29–03–MU (W.D.N.C. filed Feb. 9, 2006).

4. Laska, L. (Ed.) (1996, January). Pennsylvania man used garbage can bag to commit suicide. *Medical Malpractice Verdicts, Settlements and Experts*, 43.

5. Laska, L. (Ed.) (1996, February). Georgia man develops severe infection after extraction of wisdom tooth. *Medical Malpractice Verdicts, Settlements and Experts*, 8.

6. Laska, L. (Ed.) (1999, April). Failure to diagnose periodontal disease. *Medical Malpractice Verdicts, Settlements and Experts, 7.*

7. Laska, L. (Ed.) (1996, February). California woman claims she fell off treadmill during stress test and injured back. *Medical Malpractice Verdicts, Settlements and Experts, 6.*

8. Laska, L. (Ed.) (1999, April). Technician blamed for torn rotator cuff while loading patient on stretcher. *Medical Malpractice Verdicts, Settlements and Experts*, 22.

9. Laska, L. (Ed.) (1999, August). Lost MRI blamed for failure to detect blood clot, resulting in child's loss of left leg and damage to nerves in right leg. *Medical Malpractice Verdicts, Settlements and Experts, 18.*

10. Laska, L. (Ed.) (1999, August). Mammogram report put in wrong pile. *Medical Malpractice Verdicts, Settlements and Experts*, 21.

11. Milholland, K. (1994, February). Privacy and confidentiality of patient information. *Journal of Nursing Administration, 24*(2), 19–24.

12. *Id.*

13. Gobis, L. (1994, September). Computerized patient records: Start preparing now. *Journal of Nursing Administration, 24*(9), 15.

■ ■ ■ **Resources**

www.NurseLaw.com

Aiken, T. D. (2004). Chapter 8: Documentation and the Nurse. In: *Legal, Ethical, and Political Issues in Nursing* (2nd ed.). Philadelphia: F. A. Davis Company.

Ethical Issues

Legal and Ethical Issues Affecting Educators and Students

6

Key Chapter Concepts

- Academic Dismissal
- Arbitrary and Capricious
- District Court
- Court of Appeals
- Capriciousness
- Disciplinary Dismissal
- Due Process
- Fourteenth Amendment
- Liberty Relationships
- Private Academic Institution
- Property Right
- Public Academic Institution
- Substantive Due Process
- Sufficient Notice
- Writ of Certiorari

Objectives

At the conclusion of this chapter, the reader will be able to:

1. Identify leading cases establishing the law for faculty and students in academic institutions.
2. Discuss how the courts determine whether an individual's constitutional rights have been violated.
3. Define key strategies to avoid ethical and legal problems in academic institutions.

■ Introduction

The onslaught of court decisions that involve all professionals suggests that educators must know their legal rights and responsibilities. Educators must be responsible for their own competence as well as the competence of their students. Educators must assure that students receive the necessary learning experiences such that they have the skills to become competent practitioners.

In a similar vein, students demand fair treatment, an education that provides the skills expected of competent professionals, and a high-quality education in return for their high tuition costs. Accountability both to and for students has become increasingly more important. This chapter addresses the rights and responsibilities of both educators and students and carefully reviews the material facts set forth in leading cases that have established the law in higher education. The law in the cases is applicable to all students in academic institutions.

Case Scenario

Allen North is a dental hygienist student in his last year of college at a state institution. He met with his adviser several times, who informed him, in writing and orally, that his clinical skills were not "up to par." His adviser stated on one occasion that "if he did not improve, he was in danger of being on probation or being dismissed from the program." Allen knows that he has been having difficulty in the clinical area. He argues that his clinical instructor, Brenda South, does not "like him." Three weeks before the end of the semester, May 30, the department informed Allen that he would not graduate as expected on June 15. The department chair indicated that Allen's "clinical skills were unsatisfactory and his performance was below that of other students in his class." Allen is very upset and challenges the decision. What are the responsibilities of the chair? What are the responsibilities of the adviser and the clinical instructor? What are Allen's rights? Does he have any? What laws allow Allen to bring a lawsuit against the faculty challenging the faculty's evaluation and dismissal decision? What process is due to ensure that fairness prevails?

■ Due Process

The U.S. Constitution's **Fourteenth Amendment** protects certain individual rights from being restricted by state government. The Fourteenth Amendment mandates that no state shall deprive a person of life, liberty, or property without due process of law [1]. This provision of the amendment has been subject to great scrutiny as courts have grappled with and defined what due process is and, more specifically, what life, liberty, and property are. When considering the question of due process, it is necessary to first understand that due process protections are mandated only when a state is involved in restricting an individual's rights that the Fourteenth Amendment guarantees. The state's involvement is often referred to as **"state action"** [2]. State action, though difficult to define, is particularly relevant when addressing whether academic institutions are public (state) or private.

Public academic institutions that are affiliated with state government are deemed state institutions and are supported by state revenues. **Private institutions** are not supported by state revenues and typically receive financial support from private funding. These distinctions are noteworthy and are material in determining liability.

The U.S. Constitution limits the power of the state and federal government over faculty and students in public institutions. Private academic institutions do not have the same constraints as public institutions; however, they cannot act in a manner that is **arbitrary, capricious,** or **discriminatory** when making decisions about students and faculty. It is possible that even a private academic institution that receives state funds must abide by the due process requirements of the Fourteenth Amendment. Therefore, public or private institutions may be subject to due process requirements before **dismissing, expelling,** or **suspending** a student for academic misconduct.

■ Due Process and the Courts

In 1961 in *Dixon v. Alabama State Board of Education* [3], the court addressed the question of due process and rights of students and their relationship with the academic institution. In *Dixon,* six students at the Alabama State College for Negroes in Montgomery, Alabama, were expelled from college without notice and without a hearing for "misconduct," after they participated in several off-campus civil rights demonstrations. The students, after receiving a letter from the college president indicating that the board of education had decided unanimously to expel them, filed a lawsuit requesting that the federal district court grant them a preliminary and permanent injunction restraining the Alabama State Board of

Education and others from obstructing their right to attend college. The district court upheld the dismissals and denied the students' requests. On appeal, the U.S. Court of Appeals for the Fifth Circuit reversed the district court and remanded the case back to the circuit court for further proceedings.

The appeals court, upon reviewing the trial court's decision, held that the due process protections guaranteed in the Fourteenth Amendment required a state academic institution to give notice to students concerning their possible expulsion and provide for a hearing before the expulsion. The court also held that the following **standards** should be applied when providing notice and hearing:

1. The notice should be specific as to the charges and basis for the expulsion.
2. The nature of the hearing should be dependent on the circumstances of each case but should allow for an opportunity for both sides to present in detail their respective positions [4].

In addition, the *Dixon* court held that the students must be given the names of witnesses against them, what each witness would be testifying to, the opportunity to present their own defenses to the charges, and, if the hearing was to be held before the state board of education, a written copy of its findings and decision in the case [5].

Dixon was a leading case for students in postsecondary public academic institutions when threatened with expulsion, suspension, and/or disciplinary action. This case promulgates the idea that **fair play and due process** mandate that notice and some opportunity for a hearing are required before a student at a **tax-supported college** is expelled for misconduct. The court also reasoned that the right to notice and a hearing is so fundamental to the conduct of our society that the **waiver must be clear and explicit** [6]. Disciplinary dismissals against a student are a serious matter and can have an everlasting effect on the student's reputation and standing in the community. Without an education, students may not be able to earn an adequate livelihood or complete the duties and responsibilities of good citizens [7]. Academic dismissals are considered a serious offense.

Moreover, in 1969 the U.S. Supreme Court, in *Tinker v. Des Moines Independent Community School District* [8], recognized that school officials do not possess absolute authority over their students. Students "in" school as well as "out" of school are persons under the Constitution. They have fundamental rights that the states must respect, just as the students themselves must respect their obligations to the state [9]. In a similar vein, the U.S. Supreme Court, in *Goss v. Lopez* [10], required that all public academic institutions provide due process protections to their students. The *Goss* decision involved nine public high school students who filed a class action suit against the Columbus Board of Education and various administrators alleging that the students were all suspended without a hearing for misconduct for up to 10 days. The students alleged that the Ohio statute was unconstitutional in that it allowed a school principal to suspend a student without a hearing before the suspension [11]. The students alleged that the lack of a hearing was a violation of their procedural **due process** rights guaranteed by the Fourteenth Amendment. Accordingly, they sought to enjoin the public school officials to remove a reference to their suspension from their records [12].

The federal district court:
1. Found that the students were denied their due process rights;
2. Found that the Ohio statute permitting a suspension to occur without prior hearing, or within a reasonable time period after the suspensions, was unconstitutional; and
3. Ordered that any and all reference to the students' suspensions be removed from the school record.

The court also declared that there are **minimal requirements** that a school must undertake before a suspension is to take place. The court stated that relevant case authority would:
1. Permit immediate removal of a student whose conduct disrupts the academic atmosphere of the school;
2. Require notice of suspension proceedings to be sent to students' parents within 24 hours of the decision to conduct the proceedings;
3. Require a hearing to be held, with the student present, within 72 hours of his or her removal [13], and such a hearing should provide at a minimum
   a. Production of statements in support of the charge(s) upon which the hearing is conducted
   b. Statements by the student and others in explanation or mitigation of the student's conduct
   c. That the school permit an attorney to be present
   d. That the school should within 24 hours advise the student and his or her parents by letter of its decision and the reasons for such a decision [14].

Although the court is silent regarding the **documentation** of this process, it is important that educators document the process to create a paper trail that refutes any disparate treatment.

The defendants appealed the district court holding to the U.S. Supreme Court, and on appeal, the court affirmed the lower court's holding. Accordingly, the court held that the **property right** created by Ohio in its statute for a free public education to all residents between the ages of 5 and 21 and the state's requirement of compulsory attendance in school for an identified period of time could not be taken away, in violation of the Fourteenth Amendment requirement of due process. The court also found that because a suspension may result in damage to a student's good name or reputation among fellow students and teachers, and interfere with later opportunities for higher education and employment, the Constitution demanded that due process protections be adhered to. The Court held that some kind of notice and a hearing are necessary before a suspension takes place. This requirement is imperative in order to protect students' due process rights.

The *Dixon* and *Goss* courts addressed the question of disciplinary actions in public institutions. However, an equally compelling question is, "What are the rights of students when an academic institution dismisses a student from the program?" In 1978 the U.S. Supreme Court, in *Board of Curators of the University of Missouri v. Horowitz* [15], dealt with this question.

In *Horowitz*, Charlotte Horowitz, a former medical student, was admitted with advanced standing to the University of Missouri–Kansas City (UMKC) School of Medicine in the fall of 1971. During the final year of a student's education at the medical school, the student is required to pursue "rotational units," academic and clinical studies that pertain to various medical disciplines such as obstetrics-gynecology, pediatrics, and surgery. The **Council on Evaluation,** a body composed of both faculty and students, whose role is to recommend various actions, including probation and dismissal, evaluated each student's academic performance periodically. The **Coordinating Committee,** a body composed solely of faculty members, reviewed the council's recommendations, which the **dean** ultimately approved. Students were not typically allowed to appear before either the council or the Coordinating Committee while they reviewed students' academic performances [16].

In the spring of Horowitz's first year of study, several faculty members expressed dissatisfaction with her clinical performance during a pediatrics rotation. The faculty members noted that Horowitz's "performance" was below that of other peers in all clinical patient-oriented settings. She was also erratic in her attendance at clinical sessions and lacked a critical concern for personal hygiene. Upon the recommendation of the Council on

Evaluation, Horowitz was advanced to her second and final year on a probationary basis [17].

The faculty remained dissatisfied with Horowitz's clinical performance during the subsequent year. In fact, Horowitz's faculty adviser rated her **clinical skills as "unsatisfactory."** In the middle of the year, the council again reviewed Horowitz's academic progress and concluded that she should not be considered for graduation in June of that year. Furthermore, the council recommended that, absent "radical improvement," Horowitz **be dropped from the school** [18].

In the meantime, Horowitz was permitted to take a set of oral and practical examinations as an "appeal" of the decision not to permit her to graduate. In accordance with this "appeal," Horowitz spent a substantial portion of time with seven practicing physicians in the area who enjoyed a good reputation among their peers. The physicians were asked to recommend whether Horowitz should be allowed to graduate on schedule and, if not, whether she should be dropped immediately or allowed to remain on probation. Only two of the physicians recommended that Horowitz be able to graduate on schedule. Of the other five, two recommended that she be immediately dropped from the school. The remaining three recommended that she not be allowed to graduate in June and be continued on rotation pending further reports on her clinical progress. Upon receipt of these recommendations, the Council on Evaluation reaffirmed its prior position [19].

The council met again in mid-May to consider whether Horowitz should be allowed to remain in school beyond June of that year. Noting that the report on Horowitz's recent surgery rotation rated her performance as "low-satisfactory," the council unanimously recommended that "barring receipt of any reports that Miss Horowitz has improved radically, [she] not be allowed to re-enroll in the . . . School of Medicine" [20]. The council delayed making its recommendation official until it received reports on other rotations. When a report on Horowitz's emergency rotation also turned out to be negative, the council unanimously reaffirmed its recommendation that Horowitz be dropped from the school. The Coordinating Committee and the dean approved the recommendation and notified Horowitz of their decision. Horowitz appealed the decision in writing to the university's provost for health sciences. The provost sustained the school's actions after reviewing the record compiled during the earlier proceedings. Horowitz then sued the medical school of a public university challenging her dismissal. The U.S. District Court for the Western District of Missouri entered judgment for the university's board of curators, and the medical student appealed. The U.S. Court of Appeals [21] reversed and remanded and denied an **en banc** rehearing [22]. Certiorari was granted to the U.S. Supreme Court to consider what procedures must be accorded to a student at a state educational institution whose dismissal may constitute a deprivation of "liberty" or "property" within the meaning of the Fourteenth Amendment. The U.S. Supreme Court held the following:

1. A student who was fully informed of faculty dissatisfaction with her clinical progress and the consequent threat to her graduation and continued enrollment was accorded procedural academic due process notwithstanding the lack of a formal hearing.
2. Academic deficiency dismissals do not necessitate a hearing before a school's decision-making body.
3. The record revealed no showing of arbitrariness or capriciousness that would warrant remand of the case for consideration of deprivation of substantive due process.

The U.S. Supreme Court noted that it need not decide whether Horowitz's dismissal deprived her of a liberty interest in pursuing a medical career. They also did not have to decide whether Horowitz's dismissal infringed any other interest constitutionally protected against deprivation without procedural due process. The school fully informed respondent of the faculty's dissatisfaction with her clinical progress and the danger that this posed to timely graduation and continued enrollment. The ultimate decision to dismiss Horowitz was careful and deliberate. These procedures were sufficient under the due process clause of the Fourteenth Amendment.

▪▪▪ **What If?**

A. You learn that several students received As because they got copies of the test questions.
   1. What do you do?
   2. Is there an ethical obligation to report them?
B. You and a teacher do not get along and you can't understand why. You overhear a conversation between the teacher and her coworker that she's going to make sure you have "a rough time" because your uncle "dumped her" in college two months before the wedding. What should you do?

In *Goss v. Lopez* [23], the U.S. Supreme Court held that due process requires, in connection with the suspension of a student from public school for disciplinary reasons, that the student be given: (1) written or oral notice of the charges against him or her, (2) if denial of charges, then an explanation of the evidence, and (3) an opportunity to present his or her side of the story and to refute evidence [24]. All that *Goss* required was an informal give-and-take between the student and the administrative body dismissing him that would, at least, give the student "the opportunity to characterize his conduct and put it in what he deems the proper context" [25].

In *Goss,* the court felt that suspensions of students for disciplinary reasons have a sufficient resemblance to traditional judicial and administrative fact finding to require a "hearing" before the relevant school authority.

Academic evaluations of a student, in contrast to disciplinary determinations, bear little resemblance to the judicial and administrative fact-finding proceedings to which the full-hearing requirement is traditionally attached. In *Goss,* the school concluded that the individual students had participated in demonstrations that had disrupted classes, attacked a police officer, or caused physical damage to school property. Like the decision of an individual professor as to the proper grade for a student in his course, the determination of whether to dismiss a student for academic reasons requires an expert evaluation of cumulative information and is not readily adapted to the procedural tools of judicial or administrative decision making [26].

Even assuming that the courts can review under such a standard an academic decision of a public educational institution, no showing of **arbitrariness** or **capriciousness** was made in this case. Courts are particularly ill equipped to evaluate academic performance [27].

■ Academic Due Process

Seven years later, in 1983, a second landmark decision [28] involving academic due process and postsecondary students was made (*Regents of University of Michigan v. Ewing*). In the fall of 1975, Ewing entered the public University of Michigan's Inteflex program, a six-year program in which students earned both a bachelor's degree and a degree in medicine. A number of personal and academic problems complicated Ewing's academic performance throughout the program. After six years of being enrolled in the Inteflex program, Ewing took part 1 of the National Board of Medical Examiners (NBME) examination, which is required before students are able to enter the clinical component of the program. All medical students at the University of Michigan were required to pass the exam with a score of 345 or higher before beginning clinical rotations. Ewing received a score of 235, the lowest score ever recorded at the University of Michigan [29].

After the examination, the Promotion and Review Board unanimously voted to **drop** Ewing from the program. Ewing met with the board following his dismissal and explained the several events that gave rise to his poor performance. His mother had a heart attack, he and his girlfriend of more than five years ended their relationship, and he spent considerable time writing a paper for an essay contest. Ewing reminded the board of the time and effort he had already invested in the program and his deep desire for a career in medicine. He cited the excellent clinical work that he had done [30].

Ewing filed suit in the district court when the Promotion and Review Board did not grant his request. The district court agreed that Ewing had a **property interest** in his continued enrollment in the Inteflex program. The issue before the court was whether and to what extent academic decisions as to the qualifications of a medical student are subject to substantive due process [31]. **The test to determine a violation of substantive due process, which this court noted that it had outlined in an earlier decision [32], and which Ewing needed to establish, is that there was "no rational basis for the university's decision" or that the decision to dismiss him was "motivated by bad faith or ill will unrelated to academic performance" [33].** The district court found for the university and concluded that the university did not act in violation of Ewing's due process rights. There had been no allegations that the university's decision was based on bad faith, ill will, or other impermissible ulterior motives. The evidence demonstrated that the decision to dismiss Ewing was reached in a fair and impartial manner and only after careful and deliberate considerations [34]. "Even after a traditional substantive due process review, the court found that the evidence demonstrates no arbitrary or capricious action since the university had good reason to dismiss Ewing from the program" [35]. Moreover, the court held that Ewing did not have a contract right that required the university to give him a second chance to take part 1 of the NBME examination.

Ewing appealed the district court's ruling to the U.S. Court of Appeals for the Sixth Circuit, which agreed with the district court that Ewing had a property interest in his continued enrollment in the Inteflex program. The court held that "an implied understanding that a student shall not be arbitrarily dismissed from his university is a property interest, resting in the contractual relationship between the parties which can give rise to constitutional protections" [36]. The university argued that Ewing's dismissal was not arbitrary or capricious and cited the Medical School Bulletin that noted that the Promotion and Review Board had broad discretionary power to dismiss students who did not meet academic qualifications [37]. The appeals court reviewed the evidence and looked closely at a university document titled "On Becoming a Doctor." The pamphlet stated that "a qualified student should be given a second chance to take the NBME" [38]. Ewing did not learn of the pamphlet's contents before taking the exam, but the court noted, "this pamphlet memorialized the consistent practice of the medical school with respect to students who initially fail that examination" [39]. **The court held that "the university treated Ewing in an arbitrary and capricious manner" by not allowing him a second opportunity to take part 1 of the NBME [40].** At trial, the testimony did not determine Ewing's status as a qualified or unqualified student. Accordingly, the court of appeals reversed the decision of the district court and remanded with instructions that Ewing be allowed to retake part 1 of the NBME and be reinstated to the Inteflex program if he passed the exam [41].

The University of Michigan petitioned the U.S. Supreme Court for a **writ of certiorari** to "consider whether the court of appeals had misapplied the doctrine of substantive due process" [42]. The court considered whether the university dropped Ewing arbitrarily and agreed with the district court and the court of appeals that Ewing had a property interest in continued enrollment in the Inteflex program [43].

The court noted that the fact that the university did not permit Ewing to retake the NBME examination was not actionable in and of itself. However, the **refusal to allow Ewing to retake the examination** was important to his claim that his dismissal was arbitrary and capricious [44]. The court further noted that this is not a case in which the university's procedures were unfair or that the regents concealed nonacademic or constitutionally impermissible reasons for expelling Ewing. The district court found that the regents acted in good faith [45]. Ewing was dismissed on the basis of his entire academic record and according to procedures outlined in the university catalog.

Here the court did not find that the university deprived Ewing of his due process rights and acted arbitrarily in dropping Ewing from the Inteflex program without permitting that he retake the exam. Accordingly, the U.S. Supreme Court did not agree with the reasoning of the Court of Appeals for the Sixth Circuit that Ewing's rights were violated and therefore reversed its decision.

■ Implications for Faculty and Students

The *Horowitz* and *Ewing* decisions defined the rights to due process in academic matters on the public postsecondary campus. Students in cases since *Horowitz* and *Ewing* have claimed a **property right** in terms of admission to a program of study, continued enrollment, better grades, taking examinations, and receiving a degree [46]. In terms of **liberty relationships,** students have claimed a right to reputation or good name and the right to pursue a career [47].

Accordingly, in cases involving adverse academic decisions, all the procedural due process that is required is that students receive advance notice of the grading requirements and/or performance evaluations, specifically, notice of the academic rule. Academic rules include being informed in advance of grading policies for courses and course requirements for programs of study through such media as catalogs and syllabi, as well as being informed of performance deficiencies and negative consequences in person or in writing [48].

In the case of Allen North, the *Horowitz* and *Ewing* cases, in particular, suggest a framework for analyzing whether Allen was treated fairly. Issues to explore are whether there was sufficient notice, whether the statements made by the adviser and chair constituted notice, and whether the decision was arbitrary and capricious or careful and deliberate. In addition to these questions, it is important that students and faculty remember these key points.

Case Discussion

In *Kimberg*, plaintiff entered the School of Nurse Anesthesia as a graduate student. Plaintiff argued that paying tuition, acceptance into the program, and his matriculation created an implied-in-fact contract that required the school to comply with the student handbook. He alleged his termination violated rules and regulations for students in the program, the clinical grading policy, and daily verbal and written evaluations and procedures.

Defendant alleged plaintiff refused to communicate with regard to a demonstration that was to be performed on a mannequin and that he was not prepared for a part of the program involving the journal club. He was placed on probation even though he had 12 positive clinical evaluations. He was terminated from the program for failing to progress during an alleged probationary period.

The court:
1. Denied defendant's motion for dismissal with respect to the breach of contract claim.

2. Granted a motion for dismissal with regard to the claim for breach of covenant of good faith and fair dealing.
3. Held that due process claim issues must be addressed at trial or in a motion for summary judgment with regard to whether the parties complied with the procedural requirements and the policy of not allowing an attorney present during the hearing was not fundamentally unfair.
4. Dismissed plaintiff's claims for tortious interference with a contract claim and for punitive damages.

Source: Kimberg v. Univ. of Scranton, No. 3:06cv1209 (M.D. Pa. filed Feb. 2, 2007)

■ Conclusion

If faculty and students abide by the key points identified in this chapter, they will avoid unethical conduct and minimize the need for litigation. Courts have repeatedly held that they are not the best forum for resolving such disputes. It is up to educators to know what law is established and what should to be done to ensure that fairness is afforded to all.

■ ■ ■ Pertinent Points

1. Know your academic institution's policies on admission, dismissal, suspension, expulsion, and readmission.
2. Read your academic institution's policy statements in academic catalogs and department and/or program handbooks.
3. Follow the policy and procedures and other documents as delineated. The materials must be clear and unambiguous and state what is intended by the academic institution.
4. Know whether the academic institution has any disclaimers in its catalog or other documents giving it the right to make changes including, but not limited to, in the curriculum, course content, and other areas as it deems appropriate.
5. Establish an objective method to evaluate student, classroom, and clinical performance. *Horowitz* established that the court will not interfere with academic decision making because it is not equipped to evaluate an academic setting. Notwithstanding, the court will carefully review whether faculty decisions are any of the following:
   a. Arbitrary, capricious, malicious, and not in accordance with stated policies and procedures
   b. In bad faith
   c. Violative of the student's due process rights.

6. The court will override academic decisions if the person responsible did not exercise professional judgment and departed from accepted academic norms.
7. Provide students with a copy of the evaluation tool on the first day of class so that they are put on notice as to how they will be evaluated.
8. Evaluate the student throughout the clinical rotation. If the student is not meeting the clinical objectives, the student must be warned and told how to improve and what time constraints are placed in which to make those improvements. In addition, the student must be informed of what will happen if the improvements do not occur. For example, suspension, expulsion, dismissal, request for withdrawal, or receiving an *F* grade.
9. Grade students in accordance with stated policy.
10. Faculty must put in writing what is said to the student and include it in the student's permanent record.

■ ■ ■ Study Questions

1. What is due process?
2. Discuss the Fourteenth Amendment and how it affects the rights of students.
3. How can educators protect their university from lawsuits involving students who fail courses or clinicals?
4. What is the grievance procedure in your school?
5. Discuss when the courts may review faculty decisions.
6. Discuss your catalog and policy and procedures on admission, suspension, dismissal, and readmission.
7. Create an objective method to evaluate student, classroom, and clinical performance and present it to the class.
8. Discuss one type of evaluation tool used, its pros and cons, and how it can be changed for use in other courses.
9. In your school, what actions or inactions result in suspension, expulsion, and dismissal?
10. Select one of the cases mentioned in the readings. Determine if any newer cases have been reported on the issues tried in the case you selected.
11. Discuss one leading case that addresses a student's rights and due process.
12. Define arbitrary, capricious, and discriminatory.
13. Give examples of property rights that students may claim in a lawsuit.

14. Give examples of liberty relationships that students may claim in litigation.
15. List three key points that educators should follow when teaching students.
16. List three key points that students should know relating to admission, dismissal, suspension, expulsion, and readmission.

■ ■ ■ **References**

1. U.S. Const., amend. XIV, § 1.
2. Chandler, R., Enslen, R., & Renstrom, P. (1993). *Constitutional Law Handbook* (2nd ed.) (p. 697). Rochester, NY: Lawyers Cooperative.
3. Dixon v. Alabama State Bd. of Educ., 294 F.1ed 150 (5th Cir.), *cert. denied*, 368 U.S. 930 (1961).
4. *Id.* at 158–159.
5. *Id.*
6. *Id.* at 156.
7. *Id.*
8. Tinker v. Des Moines Indep. Cmty. Sch. Dist., 393 U.S. 503, 509 (1969).
9. *Id.* at 511.
10. Goss v. Lopez, 419 U.S. 565 (U.S. 1/22/1975).
11. *Id.* at 567, 419 U.S. 565.
12. *Id.*
13. *Id.* at 572.
14. *Id.* at 571, U.S. (1975).
15. Bd. of Curators of the Univ. of Mo. v. Horowitz, 435 U.S. 78 (1978).
16. *Id.* at 79.
17. *Id.* at 81.
18. *Id.*
19. *Id.* at 82.
20. *Id.*
21. 538 F.2d 1371 (1976).
22. 542 F.2d 1335 (1976).
23. Goss, 419 U.S. at 565 (U.S. 1/22/1975).
24. *Id.* at 581.
25. *Id.* at 584.
26. *Id.* at 583.
27. Cafeteria Workers v. McElroy, 367 U.S. 886 (1961).
28. Regents of Univ. of Mich. v. Ewing, 559 F. Supp. 791 (1983), 474 U.S. 214 (1985).
29. *Id.* at 794.
30. *Id.* at 796.
31. *Id.* at 797.
32. 435 U.S. 78 (1978).
33. *Id.* at 797.

34. *Id.* at 799.
35. *Id.* at 800.
36. 742 F.2d 913, 915 (E. D. Michigan) (1984).
37. *Id.* at 915.
38. *Id.* at 916.
39. *Id.*
40. *Id.*
41. *Id.*
42. 474 U.S. 214 (1985).
43. *Id.* at 222–223.
44. *Id.*
45. *Id.* at 224.
46. *Id.* at 225.
47. Ford, D. L., & Stope, J. L. (1986). Judicial responses to adverse academic
    decisions affecting public postsecondary institution students since
    "Horowitz" and "Ewing." *Educational Law Reporter, 110,* 517.
48. Clements v. The County of Nassau, 835 F.2d 1000 (2nd Cir. 1987).

▪ ▪ ▪ Resources

FindLaw, www.Findlaw.com
LexisONE, www.lexisone.com

Ethical Issues in Health Occupations

7

Key Chapter Concepts

- Autonomy
- Beneficence
- Bioethics
- Ethical Dilemma
- Ethics
- Justice
- Morals
- Nonmaleficence

Objectives

At the conclusion of this chapter, the reader will be able to:

1. Define morals.
2. Define a moral dilemma.
3. Define ethics and ethical dilemmas.
4. Describe moral principles that healthcare practitioners uphold in a moral dilemma.
5. List approaches to solving an ethical problem.

■ Introduction

When healthcare workers hold patients' lives in their hands, they must know the right thing to do when complications arise. Most healthcare training focuses on what steps should be taken when medical emergencies or clinically related problems arise (e.g., apply pressure to stop bleeding).

In addition to clinical and medical complications, healthcare professionals must also deal with complicated ethical dilemmas. For example, suppose the person who is bleeding is HIV positive? Or if someone did not want heroic measures taken to save his or her life, should rescue breathing be started? These are ethical dilemmas, and the healthcare worker entrusted with the well-being of patients must know—or be able to discern—what is the right and the wrong thing to do. **Ethics** is the way to decide what is the right thing to do in the case of a moral dilemma.

■ Defining Terms

What makes something right, and what makes something wrong? Usually, the answer lies in our religious, cultural, and political heritage. People have been arguing about what is right and what is wrong for thousands of years. Yet despite the variety of religions and political systems in the world, there is some agreement as to right and wrong. For example, most people believe that killing is wrong. The belief that killing is wrong is a moral belief. **Morals are ideas about right and wrong.** Killing is wrong, helping the poor is right, stealing is wrong, and easing pain is right; these are all widely shared moral ideas.

Morals should not be confused with cultural habits or customs, such as wearing certain types of clothing. Morals tend to be deeply ingrained in a culture or religion and are often part of its identity. **A moral dilemma occurs when moral ideas conflict.** The death penalty is an example of a moral dilemma. The morals in conflict are the ideas that killing is wrong and that punishing criminals is right. Many people have argued long and hard on both sides of the death penalty issue but have been unable to agree. The reason they do not agree is because two good moral ideas are in conflict, and it is not clear which "side" to take. In health care, many moral dilemmas exist. What should be done about the patient described in Case Example 7-1?

Case Example 7-1

A dental assistant is working with a dentist in the examination of a new patient. The patient has a severely abscessed tooth and will require extensive root canal work. As the assistant prepares for the invasive procedure, the patient mentions that his partner has recently died of AIDS and that he, too, has AIDS. The assistant freezes. He is afraid of getting infected with the AIDS virus. Can he refuse to assist in this procedure?

The moral dilemma in Case Example 7-1 is as follows: It is good to help people in need and it is good to protect yourself from harm. The conflict exists because the patient needs help, but by helping, the healthcare professional may be putting himself in danger by coming into contact with infected blood.

Ethics is the process of deciding what is the right thing to do in a moral dilemma. Ethics is deciding right from wrong. Ethics is about making decisions. Ethics is about acting on the basis of what is right. Ethics can be defined as declarations of what is right or wrong and of what ought to be right or wrong.

Ethics exists in all professional fields (e.g., business, journalism, politics). **Ethics that deal with patients and health care are often termed** *bioethics*. Examples include such things as end-of-life decisions, cloning, stem cell research, saving cord blood, genetic testing, surrogate motherhood, and fertility issues.

The center of health care is always the patient's need. No healthcare worker has the luxury to step back when a dilemma occurs, go home, and think about things for a while. It is also not permissible for the healthcare worker to decide that someone else with more training, knowledge, or power will figure out what to do. When the patient presents a dilemma, it is every healthcare worker's responsibility to determine what is in the patient's best interest (Case Example 7-2).

Case Example 7-2

A. A nurse's aide in a hospital is making rounds to pick up lunch trays. An elderly patient has not eaten her food, again. The aide asks if the patient wants her lunch to be heated. The patient shakes her head no. "Please just tell them I ate everything. I don't want any more food. I just want to die." The aide leaves the room with the tray but is upset. Without food, the patient will starve to death. If she lies to the nurse at the patient's request, is she helping the patient commit suicide? Can a competent adult refuse to eat? Is the patient competent?

B. You hear a physical therapist tell a patient that she will check him out of the hospital and take him home for dinner and a movie. Is this ethical or professional? Is this behavior crossing boundaries between patients and healthcare providers? Are there disciplinary or legal implications?

■ A Short History of Bioethics

Medicine had little to offer patients beyond hope, kind words, and often-unscientific treatments that held a high mortality rate until the discovery of germ theory and antibiotics in the late nineteenth and early twentieth centuries. Until then, there was little ethical debate.

Active, focused bioethical debate did not begin until this century, which saw many major medical advances. Some bioethical topics have risen, fallen, and risen again. For example, in the 1920s, euthanasia societies in the United States began the push for legalized suicide. This movement fizzled with the discovery of the extermination of the Jews and others by the Nazis in World War II. However, with all the discussion in the 1970s and 1980s of the withdrawal of life support to end suffering lives, assisted suicide has risen again as an important topic of debate in the field of bioethics. Several states have proposed legislation to legalize assisted suicide, and one, Oregon, has succeeded. **In November 1997, the Oregon Death with Dignity Act was approved, making Oregon the only state that allows physician-assisted suicide.**

Medical research is another topic of bioethical debate in this century. For example, after World War II, when it was discovered that the Nazis had performed medical experiments on Jews, there was wide agreement that medical experiments must meet certain criteria and that people must agree to serve as research subjects. And yet, in the 1960s and 1970s, it was revealed that U.S. researchers had been performing harmful experiments on African American men and disabled children without their consent. In response, committees called **institutional review boards (IRBs)** were established to review all research proposals and to ensure that all research standards were met and that research subjects were given the opportunity to understand and consent to the research. These IRBs have been in wide use since the 1970s. In the 1990s, the debate reopened on whether consent of the research subjects is always required.

The **withdrawal of life support** has been another subject of a great deal of debate in the latter half of the twentieth century. With the widespread use of intravenous (IV) solutions after World War II, Roman Catholics who operated hospitals across the United States began to debate whether IV fluids were ethically required therapy for dying patients.

Advances in medical science in the 1960s brought open-heart surgery, the first organ transplants, the first intensive care units, kidney dialysis, and cardiopulmonary resuscitation. These advancements set the stage for bioethical debates about withdrawing some of this aggressive, highly technological medical care when it did not benefit the patient. In 1970, the **right-to-die**

case of Karen Ann Quinlan appeared before the medical community. The **Harvard "brain death" criteria** were introduced, and there were fierce debates over the ethics of withdrawing life support and the very first bioethics committees evolved.

By the 1980s, the withdrawal-of life-support issues evolved into debates about **do-not-resuscitate (DNR) orders**. As in Case Example 7-2A, the withdrawal of feeding was the subject of many court cases. The use of **living wills** began to block the use of aggressive medical care before it could be started. Bioethics committees spread into hospitals in every state.

In the 1990s, the debates about the withdrawal of life support shifted slightly to focus on **assisted suicide, futile medical care, healthcare proxy, and medical durable power of attorney, and the place of economics in making decisions about expensive medical care.** Ethics committees flourished in hospitals and spread into nursing homes, hospices, and visiting nurse associations throughout the country.

Many other bioethical issues have been debated in the twentieth and twenty-first centuries as well. The national debates in the 1960s over **birth control** and **abortion** spurred ethical debate among healthcare professionals. Highly technological and expensive treatment to help **childless couples** become parents began in the 1970s with the birth of the first **"test tube" baby** and has been hotly debated ever since. **AIDS** "arrived" in the early 1980s and has been the subject of debate ever since.

▪ ▪ ▪ What If?

You hear a healthcare worker on your floor talking to a patient about adopting her baby after she delivers that evening. What are the legal and ethical implications? Are there hospital policies, procedures, or guidelines regarding this type of situation?

There is a continuing bioethical debate in the United States over how to pay for health care for the millions of people in the country who do not have healthcare insurance. Is health care a right, or is it a service that one should pay for? How much health care should Medicare and Medicaid recipients receive—a bare minimum or everything from antibiotics to expensive organ transplants?

As health care has become more complex, more technological, and more expensive, the bioethical dilemmas facing healthcare workers have become more common. Most hospital deaths now occur among patients with DNR orders, for example. Millions of Americans are not covered by any kind of health insurance, and a significant percentage of children are not up to date on required immunizations for deadly diseases. In the twenty-first century, stem cell research and cloning also head the list of debates.

All these bioethical dilemmas are realistic, daily issues in health care today. All healthcare workers will face some bioethical dilemmas in their practice (Case Example 7-3). It is important to examine these issues thoroughly. Thinking about these difficult problems ahead of time prepares the healthcare professional to deal with them in practice in order to better serve the patient.

Case Example 7-3

A certified nursing assistant has been employed by a family to take care of a seven-year-old girl severely brain damaged in a near-drowning accident when she was three. During the three months the assistant has been employed, she has gotten to know the young patient well. Although the girl cannot talk, she has learned what foods she likes and does not like, that she sleeps better if she is placed on her right side, that she cries whenever she hears loud noises, and that she likes to listen to music. One day, the nursing assistant accompanies the patient and her mother to a doctor's office for minor surgery on her hand to remove a small cyst. The doctor asks the nursing assistant to stay with the child to help hold her hand in place while the minor surgery is done. The assistant notices that the doctor is not preparing to give the child a numbing shot on her arm where the surgery is to be done. She asks about this, and the doctor states, "She doesn't need anything. She's just a vegetable."
What would you do?

■ Approaching a Bioethical Dilemma

Many bioethical dilemmas are difficult. Usually the morals that are in conflict are good moral ideas, and usually the people involved are trying to do the right thing for the patient. But still, the right thing to do is not clear. How can it be sorted out? The first move is to apply the four steps in approaching a bioethical dilemma (Box 7-1). How should the nursing assistant in Case Example 7-3 begin to solve the moral dilemma? Where should any healthcare professional begin when faced with a bioethical problem?

Box 7-1 | Approach to Bioethical Dilemma

1. **Identification:** Identify the dilemma. Which morals are involved? Which morals are in conflict?
2. **Information:** Get as much information as possible about the dilemma.
3. **Communication:** Talk with other healthcare personnel on the case. Do they think there is a dilemma too? Do they agree with your understanding of the dilemma? Talk to your supervisor.
4. **Choice:** When all the talking is done, a choice needs to be made about what to do about the dilemma. A choice *must* be made. Even choosing not to decide is to decide.

■ Steps in Resolving an Ethical Dilemma

Identify the Dilemma

First of all, the healthcare worker should **identify** that the situation is indeed a moral dilemma. Remember, morals are ideas about right and wrong. A moral dilemma occurs when two morals are in conflict. In Case Example 7-3, the morals that are in conflict are that it is right to protect your patient and that it is also right to work with other healthcare professionals to take care of the patient. Here, the nursing assistant either must be silent and allow the patient to be subjected to pain or must speak up—possibly angering the physician—in order to protect her patient. What should be done?

Obtain Information

Before anything is done, get as much **information** about the dilemma as possible. This is an essential step because often the drama or pressure of a difficult bioethical dilemma excites or intimidates people in the case. Hasty decisions may be made without all the facts. In Case Example 7-3, it would be helpful to know whether the doctor has performed minor surgery on the child before. Does he know whether she requires local anesthesia? Does this type of surgery tend to cause pain to patients?

Communicate the Dilemma

It is absolutely necessary to **communicate** about the dilemma with the people involved in the patient's care. People involved in a patient's care include everyone from other healthcare providers— nurses, doctors, physical therapists, and aides—to the patient's family or guardian. If other people do not know about the bioethical dilemma, they cannot do anything to help resolve it. In Case Example 7-3, the nursing assistant must tell the doctor that, according to her observations, the patient may be able to experience pain. It is essential that the doctor know this. The doctor may be basing his judgment about the patient on her chart and not on his direct knowledge and examination of her. If the doctor has an office nurse or a medical technician, the nursing assistant should talk to him or her about her concerns as well. If this does not alter the doctor's approach, then she also needs to communicate her concerns about the patient's potential pain to the patient's mother.

Choose the Appropriate Action

At this point, after the dilemma is identified, the information gathered, and the communication done, a **choice** must be made. Two morals are in conflict. In Case Example 7-3, the moral conflict is between protecting the patient and working with the doctor. Which is more important? On the one hand, the nursing assistant may be reluctant to anger the physician by insisting that the patient can feel pain, and she may feel that she must protect her job by remaining silent. She may reason that by protecting her job, she will be able to do more good in the long run by helping other patients in the future. On the other hand, her patient is in need of protection, and she is the one with the knowledge to protect her. In fact, it is her job to protect the patient.

▪ ▪ ▪ What If?

A patient is whisked to the operating room for emergency surgery. A coworker says she doesn't understand why they are trying to save him because he has an advance directive. What should you tell her about emergency situations and advance directives? Under what circumstances at your facility are living wills "null and void" and not followed or enforced by the healthcare providers?

■ Bioethical Principles

To assist medical professionals in making a choice, several moral principles have been identified that are important to health care. All bioethical dilemmas should be evaluated with these principles in mind.

Respect for Autonomy

To be autonomous means to have self-governance or to function independently. *Auto-* comes from a Greek word that means "self." Respect for autonomy in bioethical terms means to have respect for the patient to make his or her own decisions about what is best.

Respect for autonomy is an important principle in bioethics. In the United States there is great respect for individual rights, and the law reflects this respect. The law upholds rights of the patient to make decisions about health care. For example, patients are allowed to refuse medical treatment, even if that treatment will save their lives. Patients are not required by law to keep their doctors' appointments or to take their medicine, even if that is what the doctors, their families, and their friends think is best for them.

Current bioethical thought also reflects what has been stated in the law. Under the principle of respect for autonomy, patients should be told the truth, informed of risks and benefits of treatments, and allowed to refuse treatment.

When analyzing a bioethical dilemma, consider how the principle of respect for autonomy fits into the puzzle. Is the patient's autonomy threatened?

For example, in Case Example 7-4, the patient is a Jehovah's Witness. Ignoring her religion shows disrespect for her as an autonomous person who can choose her own religion. Lying shows disrespect because it is assumed that the patient is unable to make decisions about her medical treatment.

Case Example 7-4

A medical assistant is employed in an oncologist's office. He greets a patient he knows well, a 62-year-old woman with leukemia. Her blood work shows that her white blood cell (WBC) count is down. The assistant gives this result to the doctor, who orders an infusion of fresh frozen plasma (FFP). The assistant reminds the doctor that the patient is a Jehovah's Witness, a religious group that refuses all blood products, including FFP, in treatment. The doctor becomes angry. "Just tell her it's medicine that I ordered. Don't tell her it's a blood product. It's not red, so she'll never guess. It's the only thing I have that can help her right now." Should the medical assistant lie to the patient at the request of the doctor? Either he must obey the doctor and lie or refuse to reveal to the patient that the doctor has ordered a blood product for her, or he must disobey the doctor and inform the patient that her treatment is a blood product. His only other option is to leave the office, which will cost him his job and still not assist the patient. The medical assistant must make a choice.

Continued

Case Example 7-4—cont'd

Are the options being considered respectful or disrespectful of the patient's autonomy? What would you do? Are there potential legal implications?

Beneficence

Beneficence **means "doing good" or "being kind."** In bioethical terms, the principle of beneficence means that we, as healthcare professionals, should always try to help patients and make their situation better. Beneficence is usually the reason many people go into health care: They want to help people. It is a strong motivation behind the actions of all healthcare professionals.

When thinking about a bioethical dilemma, consider whether the actions you are considering will help the patient. For example, in Case Example 7-1, where the AIDS patient needs extensive dental work, will the dental work help the patient? Yes, it will, because he has an abscessed tooth. Will refusing to do the dental work help the patient? No, because his tooth infection could spread to other parts of his body.

Nonmaleficence

Nonmaleficence **means "doing no harm."** It is part of a physician's oath to do no harm. In bioethical terms, the principle of nonmaleficence means that healthcare professionals should avoid harming a patient. Nonmaleficence is different but sometimes overlaps with beneficence. In the case of a bioethical dilemma, it is important to make sure that the actions that you are considering do not cause the patient any harm. Nothing you do should ever make the patient worse.

In Case Example 7-3, for instance, where the doctor may do a surgical procedure on a brain-damaged patient without any anesthesia, the principle of nonmaleficence comes into play. Will performing a surgical procedure without anesthesia harm the patient? The answer is maybe, if she can feel pain. However, the pain may be short term and overall the procedure might help (the principle of beneficence) the patient.

In Case Example 7-2, where the elderly patient asked the aide to lie about how little she had eaten, the principle of nonmaleficence comes into play. Will lying for the patient harm the patient? Yes, since the patient's lack of nutrition could go unnoticed and result in deterioration, malnutrition, and possibly death.

─ ■ ■ ■ **What If?**

A patient is dying at home and changes his mind and wants
"everything done" including life-prolonging treatment. The healthcare
worker hears him but does not convey the message to the family or
physician.
1. What are the ethical implications?
2. What are the potential legal problems that can arise?

Integrity of the Health Professional

**The principle of integrity has to do with the standards of the
healthcare profession.** What sort of behavior has the profession
as a group decided to allow? What behavior is prohibited?
All professions have standards, and it is important to know
what standards apply to your profession (Case Example 7-5).

   Integrity brings to mind this question: What actions
show respect for human dignity? Lying to a patient or
refusing to provide dental care does not respect the dignity of
the patient.

Case Example 7-5

A high school student studying in a health professions course at school spends a day
following a nurse in her practice in an obstetrics-gynecology clinic. While at the
clinic, a classmate patient is treated and recognized by the student. The patient is
pregnant and is upset and unsure about what to do about her pregnancy. The nurse,
with the student watching and listening, spends a lot of time counseling the patient.
Later, another classmate stops the health professions student. "Hey, I saw you with
Didi in the clinic," the friend observes. "What was she in for? Is she pregnant?"
Should the health professions student reveal the patient's diagnosis? What are the
potential legal implications?

Justice

The principle of justice means treating everyone fairly.
Distributing health care justly or fairly is a key issue in many
ethical debates. Should health care be given to everyone or only to
those who can pay? Should more health care be given to those who
can pay and less to those who cannot? Should large amounts of
healthcare money be given for high-tech treatments for dying

patients, and should less money be given to preventive care, such as prenatal care and immunizations? Is it fair to charge more for health care for those patients who engage in poor health behaviors such as smoking, eating high-fat foods, and not using seatbelts?

In this era of high-cost health care, the principle of justice has become an important factor in bioethics. For example, in Case Example 7-1, in which the AIDS patient needs dental care, the principle of justice seems to dictate that the healthcare professional treat him the same as any other patient.

■ Conclusion

Bioethical dilemmas are not easy. Any moral dilemma poses a hard choice between two or more difficult options. At times, the healthcare professional may feel overwhelmed by what may feel like a no-win situation. It is a professional obligation, however, to attempt to determine a solution to the dilemma to try to serve the patient to the best of the healthcare professional's abilities. Following the steps outlined in this chapter will enable a professional to begin to analyze bioethical dilemmas.

■ ■ ■ Study Questions

1. What are professional ethics?
2. Define *bioethics*. Discuss a bioethical dilemma that you have read about or have encountered in practice.
3. Obtain a copy of your code of professional ethics and discuss it with the class.
4. Define and discuss the resolution process for an ethical dilemma.
5. List and define five bioethical principles.
6. Find an ethical case in literature or on the internet and do a case-study analysis.
7. Create an ethical dilemma and role-play in the class.
8. Find a bioethical issue in recent newspaper articles and discuss.
9. List three citations for bioethical resources.
10. Discuss an ethical dilemma you were faced with and how you handled it.

11. Discuss the Oregon Death with Dignity Act and the statistics regarding those who have selected assisted suicide to end their lives.
12. **Bioethical Issues:** Discuss and update the class on the issues related to (a) cloning, (b) stem cell research, (c) saving cord blood, and (d) genetic testing to determine predisposition for medical diseases or conditions.

■ ■ ■ **Resources**

Aiken, T. (2004). *Legal, Ethical, and Political Issues in Nursing* (2nd ed.). Philadelphia: F. A. Davis Company.

Anronheim, J. C. (2000). *Ethics in a Clinical Practice* (2nd ed.). Gaithersburg, MD: Aspen Publishers.

Beauchamp, T. L. & Childress, J. F. (1994). *Principles of Biomedical Ethics* (4th ed.). New York: Oxford University Press.

Beauchamp, T. L. & Walters, L. (1994). *Contemporary Issues in Bioethics* (4th ed.). Belmont, CA: Wadsworth Publishing Co.

Choice in Dying, 1035 30th St. NW Washington, DC 20007. Tel.: (202) 338–9790 and (800) 989–9455.

Cohen C. B. (Ed.) (1998). *Casebook on the Termination of Life-Sustaining Treatment and the Care of Dying.* Bloomington: Indiana University Press.

Crigger, B.-J. (1999). *Cases in Bioethics: Selections from the Hastings Center Report* (3rd ed.). New York: Bedford Books.

The Hastings Center (1987). *Guidelines on the Termination of Life-Sustaining Treatment and the Care of the Dying.* Briarcliff Manor, NY: The Hastings Center.

Hemlock Society, www.compassionandchoices.org.

Howell, J. H., Sale W. F. & Callahan, D. (Eds.) (2000). *Life Choices: A Hastings Center Introduction to Bioethics* (2nd ed.). Washington, DC: Georgetown University Press.

Jonsen, A. R., Veatch, R. M. & Walters, L. (Eds.) (2000). *Source Book in Bioethics: A Documentary History.* Washington, DC: Georgetown University Press.

Ridley, A. (1998). *Beginning Bioethics: A Text with Integrated Readings.* New York: Bedford Books.

Veatch, R. M. (1999). *The Basics of Bio-ethics.* Saddle River, NJ: Prentice Hall.

UNIT III

Common Areas of Liability and Litigation

8

Legal and Ethical Considerations in Medical Imaging

Ruth Ann Ehrlich

Key Chapter Concepts

- Angiography
- American Registry for Diagnostic Medical Sonography (ARDMS)
- American Registry of Radiologic Technologists (ARRT)
- Certified Nuclear Medicine Technologist (CNMT)
- Computed Tomography (CT) Scan
- Contrast Agent
- Contrast Media
- Echocardiography
- Flouroscopy
- Limited X-Ray Machine Operator (LXMO)
- Magnetic Resonance Angiography (MRA)
- Magnetic Resonance Imaging (MRI)
- Magnetic Resonance Mammography (MRM)
- Medical Images
- Medical Imaging Methods
- Medical Imaging Technologists
- Nuclear Medicine
- Nuclear Medicine Technology Certification Board (NMTCB)
- Plain Film Radiography
- Position Emission Tomography (PET) scan
- Radiation Exposure
- Radiology
- Registered Diagnostic Cardiac Sonographer (RDCS)
- Registered Diagnostic Medical Sonographer (RDMS)
- Registered Physician in Vascular Interpretation (RPVI)
- Registered Vascular Technologist (RVT)
- Single Proton Emission Computed Tomography (SPECT) Scan

Sonography
Ultrasound

Objectives

At the conclusion of this chapter the reader will be able to:

1. Describe, compare, and contrast the following imaging modalities:
   a. Radiography
   b. Fluoroscopy
   c. Computed tomography (CT)
   d. Magnetic resonance imaging (MRI)
   e. Sonography
   f. Nuclear medicine
2. Name three organizations that certify qualifications of medical imaging technologists and discuss the significance of proper credentials for performing medical imaging procedures.
3. List basic principles of ethics that apply to medical imaging personnel.
4. Explain the rights and responsibilities of healthcare institutions with respect to the ownership and lending of medical images.
5. Identify potential risks associated specifically with the performance of various types of imaging procedures.
6. Identify intentional torts and types of negligence that may occur in the performance of medical imaging procedures.

■ Introduction

An assortment of laws and regulations apply specifically to the creation and management of medical images. Most of these rules originate and are enforced at the state level, usually through the department of state government that is concerned with health matters. They vary considerably from state to state. Allied health professionals who perform medical imaging procedures are subject to the rules that apply specifically to their imaging duties, such as the safe use of ionizing radiation and limitations on their practice in keeping with their qualifications.

   Medical imaging technologists are responsible for a considerable degree of patient care and for the management of certain medical records, including images. Some administer medication as well. They are subject to the same laws, ethics, policies, and procedures that apply to many others with similar responsibilities.

<hr>

Case Scenario

Marcia Logan, RT (ARRT), was preparing Mr. Samuel for a fluoroscopic X-ray examination of his lower intestine, also called a barium enema study. Soon after Marcia inserted the enema catheter into Mr. Samuel's rectum, he showed signs of distress. When Marcia asked whether he was all right, he did not respond. Marcia called the radiologist, Dr. Garcia, who was in his office two doors down the hall. Dr. Garcia came immediately, took an intravenous catheter, and prepared to start an IV line for medication administration. He shouted to Marcia to get a bag of normal saline solution for intravenous infusion.

Marcia opened a drawer in the emergency cart and looked for the normal saline solution, but did not see any. She did, however, find several bags of a glucose solution that also contained medication. She handed one of these to Dr. Garcia and said, "This is D5W with lidocaine (a heart medication). Is that OK?" Dr. Garcia did not answer. He proceeded to hang the solution bag on an IV pole and connect it to the IV catheter in Mr. Samuel's arm. Within a few seconds, Mr. Samuel became unconscious and suffered a seizure.

Although Mr. Samuel eventually recovered, he sustained brain damage and was not able to return to a normal life. Mr. Samuel sued the hospital, Dr. Garcia, and Marcia Logan. Who was at fault? Could Marcia have prevented Mr. Samuel's injury? What should she have done? Who breached a standard of care? What are the legal and professional implications?

<hr>

■ Medical Imaging Methods

Radiography

Radiography refers to the process of making anatomical images using X-rays, a form of ionizing radiation. Radiography is the familiar procedure of "taking an X-ray." Bony structures can be imaged using X-rays alone; this is called **plain film radiography.** Soft tissues and hollow organs often require the use of a **contrast medium** for adequate visualization. A **contrast agent** is a substance that absorbs radiation to a different degree than the tissues being radiographed and imparts a distinctive appearance to structures that might otherwise appear the same as their surroundings. Radiographic contrast agents include gases, such as air and carbon dioxide; barium sulfate, which is commonly used for examinations of the gastrointestinal tract; and various iodine compounds that may be injected into veins, arteries, or specific organs by means of needles or catheters. *Angiography* is the term for X-ray examinations of blood vessels using special X-ray equipment and iodine contrast agents.

Case Discussion

In *Stanley,* a radiologist evaluated a chest X-ray of a nurse as part of a preemployment tuberculosis screening. His report stated the X-ray showed abnormalities including "a small nodule overlying the right sixth rib." A company policy required the prospective employer to notify the nurse (prospective employee) of the results within 72 hours, which was not done. Ten months later she was diagnosed with lung cancer.

   Did the radiologist evaluating a chest X-ray for a preemployment tuberculosis screening owe a duty of care to the prospective employee nurse to inform her or make her aware of the abnormal X-ray? Yes, despite the absence of a doctor-patient relationship, he should have acted to make her aware of the abnormality that was potentially life threatening.

Source: Stanley v. McCarver, No. CV-03-0099-PR (D. Ariz. filed June 29, 2004).

Fluoroscopy

Fluoroscopy is the use of special equipment that permits direct viewing of X-ray images in real time. It is often used in conjunction with radiography. X-ray studies of the gastrointestinal tract and the spinal canal are fluoroscopic/radiographic procedures. Fluoroscopy provides guidance for catheter placement in angiography as well as localization of instrumentation for various diagnostic and therapeutic procedures. Mobile fluoroscopes are used to visualize internal structures during surgery.

Computed Tomography (CT)

Another imaging modality that involves the use of X-rays is **computed tomography,** or CT scan. This technique was formerly termed **computed axial tomography, or CAT scan**. It produces cross-sectional slicelike images that a computer can reconstruct to display the anatomy in any plane. The most common CT studies are scans of the brain, chest, and abdomen, but this modality can be used to produce images of all parts of the body. Iodine contrast media are often injected and/or ingested in conjunction with CT scans.

Magnetic Resonance Imaging (MRI)

Magnetic resonance imaging, or MRI, is a computerized scanning method that does not involve X-rays. A powerful magnetic field and pulses of radio waves provide the energy for this modality. MRI is very commonly used to study the brain, the spinal cord, the knee, and the shoulder, but other parts of the body are examined by this method as well. For example, **magnetic resonance angiography (MRA)** is the term for MRI studies of the circulatory system, and **magnetic resonance mammography (MRM)** is used to study the breast.

Sonography

Sound waves beyond the frequency detectable by the human ear are referred to as **ultrasound**. Ultrasound technology has both therapeutic and diagnostic applications. Diagnostic ultrasound imaging, also called **sonography,** is familiar because of its application to fetal imaging during pregnancy, but ultrasound is also used to study soft tissues of many other parts of the body, particularly the contents of the abdominal and pelvic cavities and the breast. Doppler ultrasound technology is used to study the circulatory system and ultrasound guidance is used for interventions that treat pathology of the veins. **Echocardiography** is the term for ultrasound studies of the heart.

Nuclear Medicine

Nuclear medicine is the science that uses radioactive materials for diagnostic purposes. After radionuclides are injected intravenously, they are taken up in specific anatomic areas and are traced and recorded by a scanner called a **gamma camera** or **scintillation camera.** These procedures provide information about both the structure and function of the brain, the thyroid gland, the liver, the lungs, and various other organs. **Positron emission tomography (PET) scans** are sophisticated nuclear medicine procedures that involve the use of special radionuclides and a computerized scanner. **Single proton emission computed tomography (SPECT)** is similar to PET imaging but uses somewhat different equipment and unique radionuclides.

■ Credentials and Practice Requirements

Various aspects of medical imaging may require different qualifications and credentials. The use of X-rays is the most highly regulated aspect of medical imaging because of public concern over potential radiation hazards. Other imaging procedures, however, may require a high degree of skill and professional preparation. Licensing and other forms of certification help ensure quality imaging and competent patient care.

The **American Registry of Radiologic Technologists (ARRT)** is a professional organization that provides examination and certification of medical imaging technologists who are qualified by education. An ARRT certificate confers the right to use the title **Registered Technologist** and its abbreviation, **R.T. (ARRT),** in connection with the holder's name as long as the registration of the certificate is in effect. The ARRT offers primary certification in radiography (R), radiation therapy (T), and nuclear medicine (N). Postprimary specialty examinations and certifications are available in computed tomography (CT), magnetic resonance imaging (MR), mammography (M), cardiovascular interventional technology (CV), quality management (QM), sonography (S), vascular sonography (VS), and bone densitometry (BD). Certification by ARRT is nationally recognized as the standard qualification to practice radiography and is required for employment in this field by most accredited institutions. The ARRT also certifies radiology assistants, who then use the title **Registered Radiologist Assistant** and its abbreviation **R.R.A. (ARRT**). More information about ARRT and its certification programs is available at the website **www.arrt.org.**

Beyond the voluntary certification by ARRT discussed above, 41 of the 50 states have laws requiring a license or permit to apply ionizing radiation (X-rays) to humans. All states accept certification by ARRT as adequate qualification. In addition, 21 of the states recognize lesser qualifications for a limited scope of X-ray practice. Holders of these credentials are called limited X-ray machine operators (**LXMOs**), and are sometimes referred to as **practical radiographers or X-ray technicians.** The ARRT and many states have continuing education requirements for the renewal of registration, certification, licenses, or permits.

Dental radiography methods differ significantly from those used in medical radiography. Education and certification in dental radiography are usually included in the process of becoming qualified as a dental assistant or a dental hygienist. States vary in the ways they recognize such certification, and some require additional education, testing, and/or certification.

There are also separate organizations for primary certification in nuclear medicine and ultrasound technology. The **Nuclear Medicine Technology Certification Board (NMTCB)** provides examination and certification for nuclear medicine technologists, who use the letters **CNMT (certified nuclear medicine technologist)** after their names. More information about this certification can be found at the NMTCB website, www.nmtcb.org.

The **American Registry for Diagnostic Medical Sonography (ARDMS)** provides the following technologist certifications: **RDMS** (registered diagnostic medical sonographer), **RDCS** (registered diagnostic cardiac sonographer), and **RVT** (registered vascular technologist). The ARDMS also offers **RPVI** (registered physician in vascular interpretation) certification to qualified physicians. The website address for this organization is *www.ardms.org*.

The states have differing regulations regarding requirements for credentials and restrictions on the scope of practice in medical imaging. In most cases these regulations govern specifically the application of ionizing radiation to human beings. In addition, the Joint Commission on Accreditation of Healthcare Organizations (JCAHO) requires certain qualifications for technologists and supervisors in healthcare facilities who wish to be accredited. For these reasons, imaging technologists, like all healthcare workers, have a duty to be fully aware of the qualifications needed for the positions they seek and to be familiar with the permitted scope of practice for their positions in their geographic areas and in their workplaces.

There may be specific requirements beyond a license or permit. For example, the state of Washington requires blood-borne pathogen training, and many healthcare organizations require that personnel who provide direct patient care have current certification in CPR. In states where imaging technologists are permitted to administer medications and/or contrast media, there may be training requirements associated with medication administration, controlled substances, and intravenous injection procedures.

Credentials must be current and practice must meet all regulatory standards. Practicing outside these legal boundaries is usually considered a misdemeanor that may lead to fines and/or imprisonment. Employers may be held liable for illegal practice by their employees. Falsification of credentials, or fraudulent, false, or deceptive statements on applications for credentials, may lead to prosecution by the credentialing agency for fraud or misrepresentation. Conviction, pleading guilty, or pleading no contest to felony or misdemeanor charges related to providing health care are grounds for sanctions by certifying and licensing agencies. Sanctions may include permanent or temporary ineligibility for certification, revocation of certification, suspension of certification, censure, or reprimand.

It is important to be aware of the definition of practice in your area. For example, some employers incorrectly assume that they can hire nonqualified personnel to work in X-ray imaging departments as long as a qualified person actually makes the exposure. Usually, the practice of radiologic technology is legally defined to include positioning patients, positioning X-ray tubes, positioning film or other image receptors, and setting the exposure controls.

▪▪▪ What If?

You learn that a coworker has falsified his credentials and is not qualified or trained for the position. What do you do? What are the potential legal and professional implications?

▪▪▪ What If?

Louisa Martin is a medical assistant in Portland, Oregon. She has been summoned to a hearing to show cause why she should not be charged with "practicing radiologic technology without a license." When the radiation control officer made an unannounced visit to Dr. Whitfield's medical office, Louisa was in the X-ray room with a patient. The patient was lying on the X-ray table and Louisa was manipulating the dials on the X-ray control panel.

Louisa testifies that she did not practice radiologic technology. "I never pushed the button," she said. "I would prepare the patient and the room for the examination, and then Dr. Whitfield would come by the room and make the exposure."

Louisa is guilty of practicing radiologic technology illegally because Oregon Administrative Rules state: "The 'Practice of Radiologic Technology' shall be defined as but not limited to the use of ionizing radiation upon a human being for diagnostic or therapeutic purposes including the physical positioning of the patient, the determination of exposure parameters, and the handling of the ionizing radiation equipment." What are the legal and ethical implications?

Ethics

The codes of ethics of professional organizations in the imaging field have provisions similar to those found in other codes for healthcare professions. They include providing quality care with respect for patient dignity and without discrimination on any basis. They require that privileged communication must not be revealed except as permitted by law. They prohibit practice when there is actual or potential inability to practice safely due to illness, the use of alcohol or drugs, or any physical or mental condition. They promote adherence to scientific principles and accepted procedures. Radiologic technologists are held to a standard of expertise in minimizing radiation exposure to patients, to themselves, and to other members of the healthcare team. They are not allowed to diagnose, holding this to be the responsibility of physicians. They are expected to conduct themselves professionally.

The **Standards of Ethics of the ARRT** is a document made up of two parts: The Code of Ethics is an aspirational document consisting of 10 principles, and the Rules of Ethics lists prohibited practices that are enforceable by sanctions. (See **www.asrt.org/media/pdf/codeofethics.pdf.**)

▪ ▪ ▪ What if?

You are a radiographer and are working the late shift. You are called to the emergency room to take X-rays of an injured wrist. You see what appears to be a fracture through the distal end of the radius, but when you show the images to Dr. Harcourt, the ER physician, she says, "Just as I thought—perfectly normal." The radiologist is out for the evening and will not see the films until morning. According to ASRT Code of Ethics, you are prohibited from making a diagnosis. What should you do?

Medical Images

All medical images, made in all modalities and using all types of media (film, paper, videotape, CD-ROM, electronic, and digital files), are considered part of the patient's legal medical record. They are subject to HIPAA (Health Information Portability and Accountability Act) requirements for privacy and are the property of the institution in which they originate, although the patient has the right to obtain a copy of his or her medical records.

Legal requirements for the retention of medical images vary from state to state and may differ from the retention requirements for other medical records. In most cases, the retention period for the records of minors begins when the patient reaches the age of majority. This age also differs from one state to another. Consider this example: In a state where the retention period for records is five years, and the age of majority is 18 years, the records must be maintained until the patient has reaches the age of 23, five years after reaching majority. This practice gives patients access to their childhood medical records for a reasonable period after they become adults. For this reason, film files and electronic records on minors are tagged so that they will not be discarded when the usual minimum retention period for adults has elapsed.

In major imaging centers and large medical facilities, medical images are made in digital format or converted to a digital signal for storage. The combination of hardware and software used to store, manage, copy, transmit, and manipulate these images, and to associate them with the pertinent patient information, is called a **picture archiving and communication system,** often referred to by the acronym **PACS**. In the future, all medical images will probably be in digital format, but these systems are presently too expensive to be feasible for small hospitals and clinics and for physicians' offices. While there is a major trend in the direction of digital formats for all medical imaging, in smaller facilities X-ray images are still recorded and stored on film.

It is often desirable for healthcare institutions to share medical images with other health professionals who are providing care to the patient. In the case of digital images, all copies are identical and the PACS can easily provide either full-size film copies or CD-ROM files when there is a need to share images with others. X-ray films can be copied also, but the copies are not equal in quality to the original images. For this reason, the original films are often loaned directly to other healthcare providers.

When medical images, originals or copies, are sent to another provider for the patient's benefit, the patient must sign a release form permitting the transfer. A dated record must be kept of the name and location of the person or institution that receives the images. If original images are sent out and then subpoenaed by the court, the legal requirement to produce the images is satisfied by producing the record of the name and address of the person to whom they were sent and the date of the loan.

▪ ▪ ▪ **What if?**

> You see a physician take an X-ray film that is later determined to be an important piece of evidence in a medical malpractice case (and is now "lost"). What are the legal and ethical issues?

■ Risks Related to Imaging Procedures

Imaging professionals have a duty to understand potential hazards to their patients and to take appropriate precautions to prevent injury. Failure to do so is negligent and may cause harm to the patient for which the healthcare worker could be liable.

Ionizing Radiation

Radiation exposure is an imaging hazard. The public is generally aware that X-rays may be harmful. In fact, the risk of injury from routine diagnostic studies is extremely small. The chance of death as a consequence of X-ray exposure from a chest X-ray, for example, is less than one in a million. On average, life-span shortening to the general population as a result of diagnostic X-ray exposure is less than six days. Most X-ray examinations expose the patient to much less radiation than the average amount received by the population from natural background exposure every year.

Cancer and leukemia are the principal random, unpredictable effects that occur as a result of exposure to low doses of X-rays. These effects are not immediate. They manifest themselves anywhere from 5 to 30 years after exposure; they also occur in the absence of exposure. These effects are apparent as statistical phenomena, but it is not possible to associate a low radiation dose with any effect in any one individual.

The potential for negative effects of radiation exposure during pregnancy poses a somewhat greater concern. The risk is minimal when the dose to the maternal abdomen is less than 5 rad (0.05 Gray), an amount equal to more than 10 times the average diagnostic X-ray exposure. However, multiple examinations, particularly CT examinations of the abdomen or pelvis, may result in a total dose that is sufficient to cause concern.

During the first two weeks following conception, the greatest risk is the possibility of spontaneous abortion (miscarriage). During weeks 3 through 14, exposure to the embryo poses a risk of abnormal development. Birth defects such as spina bifida, cleft palate, and neurological abnormalities may result from exposure during this period. Once the fetus is fully formed, radiation exposure may still be detrimental. Research has demonstrated a higher incidence of premature birth, low birth weight, and childhood cancer among children irradiated in utero.

Contrast Media

A great variety of **contrast media** is available for X-ray imaging of various parts of the body. While these agents are considered quite safe, they may be hazardous to certain patients who have high risk factors. The patient's medical history must be checked to screen for risk factors. For example, patients with certain **heart** conditions may be at risk from **iodine** injections, and patients with **kidney** disease or kidney failure cannot eliminate iodine products effectively. There is also risk of kidney complications when iodine compounds are administered to **diabetic** patients who are taking certain medications to control hyperglycemia.

When iodine compounds are injected into the circulatory system for studies of the blood vessels or the urinary tract, there is risk of a severe allergic reaction called *anaphylaxis*, which may be life threatening. These risks have been minimized by the development of **nonionic contrast agents**. A patient's allergy history is the most accurate predictor of the likelihood of such a reaction. Emergency supplies are kept at hand to respond to such an occurrence and personnel are trained to recognize the onset of an allergic reaction and respond appropriately. Such events are rare.

Other risks associated with the administration of contrast media include **extravasation of the medium into the tissues** surrounding the vein during an intravenous injection. This condition is very uncomfortable and may cause significant damage to the tissues if not treated promptly. The possibility of extravasation is of particular concern during large-volume intravenous injections by automatic injectors during CT scans.

MRI Scans

There is no ionizing radiation involved in MRI imaging. The magnetic fields and radio waves used in this modality do not produce any documented side effects that are significant. Although no adverse effects have been reported as a result of MRI during pregnancy, these procedures are generally avoided in the first 12 weeks of pregnancy. The risks associated with MRI imaging fall into four basic categories: **(1) oversedation, (2) allergic reaction to contrast agent gadolinium, (3) injury caused by the action of the magnetic field to metal or electronic devices within the body, and (4) thermal injury.**

Many MRI gantries are tubular structures in which the patient is confined during the procedure. This can cause a **claustrophobic response** that is often treated by the intravenous administration of a tranquilizing medication such as diazepam. MRI scans often require the patient to be absolutely still during the several minutes required for each scan sequence. When pain patients are unable to hold still because of pain, narcotic medications such as meperidine or morphine may be administered to alleviate discomfort. Both tranquilizers and narcotic analgesics may cause **respiratory depression** leading **to respiratory arrest** if the dosage is beyond the limits tolerable to the patient. To ensure the safety of sedated patients during MRI procedures, technologists monitor their pulse rate and the oxygen saturation levels in their blood by means of a pulse oximeter attached to the patient's finger or earlobe.

Gadolinium compounds are the type of intravenous contrast agent used for MRI imaging and are considered very safe. There have been documented **allergic reactions** to gadolinium, but these are extremely rare. Of somewhat greater concern is a recent FDA notice advising of a link seen between the use gadolinium compounds in relatively high doses for MRA and a disease called **nephrogenic systemic fibrosis, or nephrogenic fibrosing dermopathy (NSF/NFD)** that occurs in patients with kidney failure. This underscores the need for **careful history-taking** and **screening of patients** who are given *any* medication and particularly contrast media.

Patients and all other persons entering the MRI scan room must be screened for **metal** objects. The powerful magnetic field surrounding the scanner attracts **metal objects** containing iron or steel, sending them flying through the air and into the bore of the magnet. **Serious injuries are caused when scissors, oxygen tanks, magnetic wheelchairs, and other metallic objects are brought into the magnetic field.** It is important to note that the magnetic field is present even when the scanner is idle.

In addition to metal objects brought into the room, patients must be screened for possible **magnetic metallic objects in their bodies** because the magnetic field may cause these foreign bodies to move, causing injury. When a careful history cannot rule out the possibility of metallic foreign bodies in the soft tissues, patients may be screened by CT scan prior to the MRI study. This is a particular concern with patients such as welders whose occupational activities may have resulted in metallic foreign bodies within their eyes.

While most surgical implants and orthopedic hardware are made of nonmagnetic metals that are safe in the scanner, there is risk of injury when patients with certain kinds of implants are scanned. **Pacemakers and internal cardioverter defibrillators (ICDs)** are of particular concern. MRI scanning is **contraindicated** for patients with these devices because the magnetic field may cause a device to malfunction, placing the patient at risk. In addition, thermal effects may damage the device or burn the patient. Although rare, serious injuries and fatalities have occurred as a result of scanning patients with pacemakers and ICDs. Recent developments in these devices have made them safer in magnetic fields than they once were, but further engineering development is needed before pacemakers and ICDs are considered safe for routine MRI procedures.

Patients undergoing MRI studies have sustained **second- and third-degree burns** as a result of skin contact with surface coils or monitoring cables. Although some of the reported thermal injuries have been serious enough to require skin grafts, no life-threatening incidents have been reported. These burns are preventable by ensuring that the patient's skin is not in direct contact with surface coils or gantry and that monitoring cables are not looped across the patient's body.

Nuclear Medicine Imaging

Nuclear medicine scans are usually performed primarily with a **man-made radioactive element called technetium (^{99}Tc)** that can be attached to other molecules that have an affinity for certain types of tissues or organs. Since technetium has a very short half-life, it is considered very safe, both for the patient and for those who care for the patient. The practice of using **radioactive iodine (^{131}I)** for whole body scans results in a greater radiation dose and is therefore contraindicated for women who are pregnant and for those who are nursing.

Diagnostic Ultrasound

The Food and Drug Administration (FDA) reports that ultrasound is a form of energy that laboratory studies have shown can produce physical effects in tissue, such as jarring vibrations and a rise in temperature, even at low levels. For this reason it cannot be considered completely innocuous. There are, however, no known harmful effects to humans associated with any diagnostic ultrasound procedure, and sonography is considered a very safe procedure for obtaining information about pregnancy.

■ Torts Related to Imaging

During many imaging procedures, the technologist is the only healthcare professional present with the patient. For this reason, these technologists are trained in patient care and are subject to the same types of risks and liabilities as other healthcare personnel who provide direct care.

Intentional Torts

Among the **intentional torts** that can be attributed to imaging personnel are **assault, battery, false imprisonment, libel, slander, fraud, invasion of privacy, misrepresentation, and the intentional infliction of emotional distress.** For example, performing a procedure on the wrong patient or continuing a procedure after the patient has withdrawn consent may constitute grounds for a charge of battery. Improper use of restraints might be cause for a charge of false imprisonment.

Negligence

Negligence may be charged when patients are injured due to falls or extravasation of contrast media. **Medication errors** are a potential source of litigation that may involve imaging technologists who assist with medication administration. **Accurate, validated communication and proper documentation** are essential to refuting defensible charges of negligence. Those with professional qualifications, such as certification by ARRT or ARDMS, are considered capable of independent judgment within the scope of their job descriptions. They are responsible and liable for the decisions they make. This may be true even in cases where the employer is found to be liable as well. They are held to the standard of the reasonable technologist in similar circumstances.

In the scenario at the beginning of this chapter, Mr. Samuel was allegedly harmed by the negligence of Dr. Garcia and Marcia Logan. In hindsight, it is clear that it would have been preferable for Marcia to continue looking for normal saline solution and to have left the other solution in the emergency cart. In fact,

Dr. Garcia was at fault for failing to read the label on the solution before connecting it to the IV line. Marcia had a professional duty to be familiar with the locations of emergency supplies. She also failed to communicate effectively with Dr. Garcia. When he did not respond to her question, her communication was not validated. She had a duty to make certain she had been understood. This incident illustrates how easily assumptions and miscommunications can cause problems, especially in the emotionally charged urgency of emergency situations.

Lawsuits have been brought against imaging technologists as a result of **missed diagnosis due to poor quality of images.** While this is a rare occurrence, it highlights the need for professional competence and ethical decision making in the clinical setting.

Invasive procedures such as angiograms require that the patient provide **informed consent. Imaging technologists have a duty to be aware of what procedures require this formal consent and who is authorized to obtain the consent.** They must check for the presence of the signed consent before proceeding with any procedure that requires it. Those who obtain consent must be thoroughly familiar with the procedure and able to explain the material risks that may be involved. Failure to obtain the required consent may lead to liability for assault, battery, or misrepresentation.

Imaging personnel use patient charts and institutional computers to obtain information about their patients, to check orders, and to enter data about procedures. While information provided to imaging technologists is not considered legally privileged, it may be so considered when they are acting on behalf of a physician. Because they have access to confidential information, they are obligated, both ethically and legally, to maintain the confidentiality of such information.

■ Conclusion

Medical imaging is performed principally by professional technologists who are educated, certified, and/or licensed to provide imaging services and patient care. They are bound by the broad principles of medical ethics, specific professional standards, and the laws that govern radiation use, medication administration, patient care, and medical records. As members of the healthcare team, they are held to high standards of competence, patient care, and professional judgment.

1. *Radiography* is the term for making anatomical images using X-rays.
2. Contrast media are used to enhance visualization of anatomical structures in radiography, fluoroscopy, CT scans, and MRI scans.
3. MRI scans use a magnetic field and radio waves to generate computer images of anatomical structures.
4. In most states, specific credentials are required to perform X-rays on human beings.
5. ARRT, ARDMS, and the NMTCB are professional agencies that examine and certify technologists in various aspects of medical imaging.
6. The ethics that apply to imaging technologists include the broad principles that apply to all aspects of health care; in addition, they are required to minimize radiation exposure and are not permitted to diagnose.
7. Medical images are considered a part of the legal medical record and are subject to retention regulations and HIPAA requirements.
8. The risks of harm from radiation exposure as a result of diagnostic imaging are extremely small; the greatest radiation risk involves exposure to pregnant patients as a result of multiple relatively high-dose examinations, such as CT scans of the abdomen or pelvis.
9. The injection of iodine contrast media into the circulatory system poses the possibility of anaphylaxis, kidney failure, and heart failure to patients who are at high risk.
10. Safety practice is essential to avoid risk of injury from the magnetic field to patients receiving MRI scans.
11. Sonography is the safest imaging method used to investigate pregnancy.
12. Imaging technologists are responsible for patient care in the scope of their duties and may be liable for intentional torts or negligence if their practice is not consistent with legal and ethical standards.

■ ■ ■ **Study Questions**

1. List three imaging modalities that involve the use of X-rays.
2. What is the term for imaging methods that involve the injection of radioactive substances?

3. What aspects of a patient's medical history might be important with respect to risks associated with diagnostic imaging?
4. Who owns medical images?
5. List five principles of medical ethics that apply to imaging technologists.
6. Define *anaphylaxis* and describe the circumstances when a patient might be at risk for this condition.
7. What kinds of substances are used as contrast agents in X-ray imaging? What type is used in MRI?
8. Which imaging modality may cause thermal damage?
9. Discuss the duties of an imaging technologist with regard to medical records.
10. Describe a circumstance that might result in a charge of intentional misconduct by an imaging technologist, and one that might lead to liability for negligence.

▪ ▪ ▪ Resources

ARDMS, www.ARDMS.org.

ARRT, www.ARRT.org.

Bushong S. (2004). *Radiologic Science for Technologists*, (8th ed.). St. Louis: Mosby/Elsevier, 2004.

Joint Commission on Accreditation of Healthcare Organizations, www.jointcommission.org/Standards/.

Kalin R. & Stanton, M.S. (2005). Current clinical issues for MRI scanning of pacemaker and defibrillator patients. *Pacing Clin. Electrophysiol. 2005; 28*:326–328.

Leal Del Ojo, J., Leal, M. F., Villaba, J., et al. (2005). Is magnetic resonance imaging safe in cardiac pacemaker recipients? *Pacing Clin. Electrophysiol. 2005; 28*:274–278.

Medical Device Safety Reports, www.mdsr.ecri.org/summary/detail.aspx?doc_id=8178.

Medline Plus, www.nlm.nih.gov/medlineplus/ency/article/003335.htm.

Medscape, www.medscape.com/viewarticle/503383.

NMTCB, www.NMTCB.org.

Oregon Administrative Rules 337-010-0006, Board of Radiologic Technology, Division 10, Licensure, Definitions.

Oregon Revised Statutes, §§ 688.405–688.605

Procedural Guideline for General Imaging, National Guideline Clearing house., http://www.guideline.gov/summary/summary.aspx?ss=15&doc_id=7085&nbr=4258.

RadiologyInfo, www.radiologyinfo.org.

Statkiewicz Sherer, M. A., Visconti P., & Ritenour, E. R. (2006). *Radiation Protection in Medical Radiography* (5th ed.). St. Louis:: Mosby/Elsevier, 2006.

9

Administrative and Medical Record Liability and Litigation

Key Chapter Concepts

- Audit Trails
- Biometric Identification System
- Breach of Confidentiality
- Computer Password
- Consent
- Health Insurance Portability and Accountability Act (HIPAA)
- Intentional Tort
- Need-to-Know Exception
- Negligence
- Right of Privacy
- Subpoena
- Subpoena Duces Tecum
- Tort

Objectives

At the conclusion of the chapter, the reader will be able to:

1. Discuss the importance of protecting a patient's right to privacy.
2. Discuss the need-to-know rule.
3. Define the difference between invasion of privacy and breach of confidentiality.
4. Outline the types of discrimination that can result from the inappropriate release of patient information.
5. Discuss four types of patient information that require heightened protection.
6. Outline computer safety measures that can be taken to protect patient information.
7. Describe the circumstances that force a facility to refuse to respond to a subpoena duces tecum.

■ Introduction

Individuals who, because of the nature of their jobs, have access to and/or are responsible for maintaining patient healthcare records face many potential ethical dilemmas and legal pitfalls. Whether you are a health information technologist or administrator, a medical assistant, a medical custodian, or a medical record transcriptionist, you have access to and control of sensitive patient information. It does not matter what type of healthcare facility employs you. If such information is inappropriately accessed or released, there may be legal ramifications.

Case Scenario

Ester Levin is a health information administrator at North Island Medical Center. David Farmer, the hospital's vice president of human resources, approaches her and requests that Ms. Levin provide him with a printout of certain healthcare records pertaining to Dr. Robert Lewis. Dr. Lewis is employed as a surgical resident at the medical center and was recently hospitalized there. Rumor has it that Dr. Lewis is homosexual and may have tested positive for HIV while hospitalized.

Ms. Levin knows from her training in health information management that information about patients who are HIV positive or diagnosed with acquired immunodeficiency syndrome (AIDS) must be carefully protected. Ms. Levin does not think it appropriate to provide the requested information to Mr. Farmer. Although Mr. Farmer is responsible for hospital personnel, he has never before personally requested hospital records from the patient records department. Ms. Levin asks Mr. Farmer if he has a signed consent form from Dr. Lewis. Mr. Farmer states he does not need one as he is the director of human resources and Dr. Lewis is an employee. Ms. Levin is afraid that if she refuses to provide the requested information she could be disciplined or even lose her job. What should she do?

Failure to adhere to the principles discussed below can lead to legal liability both for the individual who inadvertently or deliberately accesses or releases confidential patient information and for the healthcare facility for which the responsible individual works.

■ Healthcare Record Liability

Why should you be so concerned about maintaining the confidentiality of a patient record? Our legal system provides each individual with the right of privacy that includes a patient's right to expect that the healthcare record will remain confidential. This right is derived from common law and constitutional law. There are reported legal decisions that uphold a patient's right of privacy, as well as federal and state statutes and regulations that protect this right. For example, hospital regulations in many states require acute care facilities to have a medical records department, which is primarily responsible for maintaining medical records for all inpatients treated at the hospital and outpatients treated at the clinics.

Protections such as these are necessary to ensure a patient's right of privacy and to prevent emotional distress from the humiliation and embarrassment of an unauthorized disclosure. Such protections also are necessary because, at times, an individual's health history leads to discrimination at work, in school, or when applying for certain types of insurance, primarily health and life insurance.

In *Robley v. Blue Cross/Blue Shield of Mississippi,* plaintiff was treated for severe deep abscesses that required continued care after discharge [1]. Because of the patient's history of migraines and her husband's concerns that he couldn't properly care for her wounds, approval was sought for a home health nurse. An employee of a wound care center called Blue Cross for approval, and a case manager at Blue Cross referred to the patient as a "drug seeker." This was relayed to the patient's husband. Plaintiff claims that upon overhearing this she entered a psychotic state, which aggravated her migraines and left her bedridden for days. She frequently became violent and annoyed and suffered bouts of crying, too. She sued Blue Cross and sought damages for intentional and negligent infliction of emotional distress as well as breach of confidentiality based on an allegation that Blue Cross had a fiduciary duty to maintain confidentiality of these records.

The Supreme Court of Mississippi held that the contract did not create a fiduciary relationship. The court also held that the trial judge erred in granting a directed verdict on the issues of breach of confidentiality and negligent infliction of emotional distress. The court reversed and remanded it for the jury's determination on those issues.

■ Right of Privacy and Consent

The right of privacy, however, is not absolute. An obvious exception to a facility's policy of nondisclosure is a patient's **consent** to the release of healthcare information. Patients may give consent for various reasons, such as providing another healthcare provider or facility with healthcare history in order to receive appropriate treatment. In addition, a patient usually is required to consent to the release of records to the health insurance carrier or managed-care company in order to obtain healthcare benefits. Often, healthcare providers are required to disclose certain patient information to governmental authorities. For example, state departments of health require that certain communicable diseases, such as tuberculosis, be promptly reported to the appropriate authorities. In various states the information submitted must contain identifying information for the person diagnosed unless the patient is tested in one of a limited number of testing sites within the state that offer state-mandated anonymous testing.

Under these types of circumstances, a state's interest in protecting the health, safety, and welfare of the public from the threat of communicable diseases outweighs the individual patient's right of privacy. Patient information that is necessary to provide appropriate patient care can be shared between and among treating healthcare providers within the same facility, but such information must not go beyond those who have a **need to know.** For example, a treating physician may order a dietary consultation for his diabetic patient who is about to be discharged from the hospital. The nutritionist is permitted access to the patient record in order to obtain certain information and make an entry regarding the consultation but is not permitted access to a record pertaining to a prior hospitalization of the same patient for a mental illness. Patient records also can be subpoenaed under certain circumstances. If the subpoena is valid, the patient's records must be released.

■ Violations of Patient's Right of Privacy

If an exception for disclosure does not exist and a patient's record is inappropriately released or accessed, that patient's right to privacy is violated. Claims against healthcare workers for **negligence** and/or **quasi-intentional torts** can follow (Box 9-1). **Invasion of privacy** and **breach of confidentiality** are the most common quasi-intentional torts alleged in lawsuits dealing with the inappropriate disclosure of patient information. *Quasi* means "resembling," and quasi-intentional torts are based on speech. (Another quasi-intentional tort is **defamation.** Defamation in the written form is **libel** and oral defamation is **slander**.)

Box 9-1 | Quasi-Intentional Torts

Invasion of privacy
Breach of confidentiality

Invasion of privacy occurs when someone who has no right to access a patient's healthcare record does so anyway, thereby intruding on the private concerns of the patient.

Breach of confidentiality occurs when someone who has legitimate access to health information about a patient shares it with others who have no need to know. For example, in *Pierce v. Caday* [2], a patient sued her healthcare provider for failure to protect her confidential information from disclosure. The healthcare provider's employees had access to the information and discussed it with others. Although the patient's lawsuit was unsuccessful, it demonstrates that such litigation occurs and affects employees of healthcare providers, such as health information management administrators and technicians, medical administrative assistants, medical transcriptionists, and medical secretaries.

Another example of the legal theories used in liability cases for improper disclosure of patient records is *Estate of Behringer v. Princeton Medical Center* [3]. In the *Behringer* case, Dr. Behringer, a physician with surgical privileges at Princeton Medical Center who was also a patient, sued for damages that resulted when the medical center and its employees breached the duty to protect the confidentiality of his diagnosis. In June 1987, Behringer became ill and was admitted to the medical center for treatment. Part of Behringer's medical workup included a bronchoscopy and a blood test for HIV. He tested positive for HIV, and the bronchoscopy confirmed the presence of *Pneumocystis carinii* pneumonia (PCP), a common condition found in AIDS patients. These two findings led to a diagnosis of AIDS. The treating physician advised Behringer of the diagnosis, and Behringer was then discharged from the hospital to be treated at home. He was concerned that his diagnosis would become general knowledge—a concern that was not unfounded.

Once home, Behringer received numerous phone calls from physicians at the medical center. The physicians were not his treating physicians and had no reason to know his diagnosis, although it was clear that they did. Approximately one month after his hospitalization, Behringer returned to his medical practice, but it was evident that many of his patients had become aware of his diagnosis and his practice began to deteriorate. He lost patients and employees, and his surgical privileges at the hospital were canceled when the chief of nursing told the president of the medical center about Behringer's diagnosis. Although Behringer wished to continue performing surgery, he was not allowed to do so. He managed to continue an office practice until his death approximately two years later.

Before his death, Behringer filed a lawsuit against the medical center and some of its employees. The lawsuit alleged, among other things, that the defendants breached their duty to maintain the confidentiality of Behringer's diagnosis. The court agreed. Although the court recognized the **need-to-know exception** to the general rule of confidentiality of patient information, it was clear that the boundaries of the exception had been violated as a result of several factors. The hospital's laboratory had failed to take adequate steps to maintain the confidentiality of the diagnostic test results. In addition, the hospital was negligent as the custodian of patient charts. It failed to take certain steps to limit access and maintain the confidentiality of the records. Although the medical center instructed its employees that medical records were confidential, it was not enough. The medical center knew that most of its staff could access any patient chart with or without authorization. The court found this unacceptable.

Fairfax Hospital v. Curtis sets forth another example of the legal theories used in such liability cases [4]. In *Fairfax*, the patient Ms. Curtis sued a hospital and two of its employees for compensatory and punitive damages. Curtis claimed that her confidential medical records were improperly released to third parties without her consent. The trial court awarded her $100,000, and the defendants appealed. The Supreme Court of Virginia upheld the award.

The facts of the case are as follows: Plaintiff Curtis was a patient at Fairfax Hospital, where she received prenatal care and eventually gave birth to a child. During her treatment, she provided certain information about herself to the healthcare providers. The court did not specify the nature of the medical information she provided (apparently to protect her from further disclosure of confidential information), but it stated that "the medical records contained very personal information about plaintiff's medical history before and after her pregnancy" [5]. After the birth, the child suffered cardiopulmonary arrest and died. Plaintiff, as the representative of the child's estate, filed a malpractice claim against the hospital. After receiving notice of the claim, the hospital released a copy of plaintiff's medical records to the attorney it had retained to defend the claim. That attorney, in turn, released the records to a defendant nurse in the malpractice case.

The defendants argued that plaintiff's medical records were properly disclosed because they were at issue in the malpractice case. The court disagreed because, at the time the hospital released plaintiff's records, it was the deceased child's medical condition at issue, not the mother's medical condition. The court determined that releasing such information without the patient's consent was a **tort:**

> [A] healthcare provider owes a duty of reasonable care to the patient. Included within that duty is the healthcare provider's obligation to preserve the confidentiality of information about the patient, which was communicated to the healthcare provider during the course of treatment. Indeed, confidentiality is an integral aspect of the relationship between a healthcare provider and a patient and, often, to give the healthcare provider the necessary information to provide proper treatment, the patient must reveal the most intimate aspects of his or her life to the healthcare provider during the course of treatment. [6]

Patients have a right to assume that if they share information with their healthcare provider, it remains confidential and is shared only for the purposes of ensuring appropriate treatment and proper recordation.

Healthcare facilities are required to implement meaningful **restrictions on access to patient records.** It is not enough that they merely instruct all employees about the confidentiality of patient information. Healthcare facilities must actively limit or prevent access in keeping with the **Need-to-Know Exception.** Failure to act accordingly can result in serious harm to the patient, as it did in the *Behringer* case. Also, those who have access to patient charts and have a right to know the information are liable for breach of confidentiality if they share it with others who have no need to know. Those that access patient charts without authorization and no right to know invade the patient's privacy. Healthcare workers must vigilantly avoid becoming involved in either situation.

■ Concerns about Computerized Patient Records

The goal of preventing inappropriate disclosure of patient information seems overwhelming today. The explosion of computer technology presents myriad challenges to healthcare workers. Most healthcare facilities now maintain all or at least a partial computerized patient record (CPR) for each patient. In addition, the recent transition from traditional forms of healthcare delivery to the present managed-care model has contributed to the challenges of the information age.

▪▪▪ What If?

A coworker takes home a hospital laptop that has confidential information on it.
1. What are the legal and ethical issues?
2. What should you do?
3. What are potential confidentiality problems that can arise?

The movement into a managed care environment and the need for data management systems in healthcare are posing new legal issues related to maintaining the privacy and confidentiality of computerized patient records. Many of these concerns are heightened as development continues toward massive patient databases that will be the primary data system for numerous networked managed care providers [7].

Unfortunately, not all federal and state laws and regulations have kept pace with the challenges that CPRs present. The federal government proposed standards to address the security, integrity, confidentiality, and availability of individual health information pursuant to the Health Insurance Portability and Accountability Act (HIPAA) of 1996, enacted by the U.S. Congress [8]. HIPAA allows for portability of group insurance coverage such that a person with a preexisting condition who has had continuous health coverage for more than 12 months can leave a job and not be declined for health insurance at the new job. Also, HIPAA includes a privacy rule that created national standards to protect patients' or clients' personal health information.

Health information management professionals and medical assistants, transcriptionists, and secretaries must be thoroughly familiar with the healthcare provider's data management system and the pertinent policies and procedures pertaining to it. They must also have some understanding of the federal and state laws and regulations that affect their job.

▪ Sensitive Types of Patient Information

There are four types of patient information that are entitled to increased protection from inappropriate disclosure due to the

sensitive nature of the information and the likelihood that it may form the basis for discrimination (Box 9-2). Patient information that contains references to the following conditions must be carefully guarded:
- Substance abuse
- Mental illness
- Sexually transmitted diseases
- Genetic makeup

Genetic makeup has become the latest area to cause concern regarding confidentiality. Scientists have the ability to detect carriers of certain diseases such as cystic fibrosis, sickle-cell anemia, and Huntington's disease. Advances in genetic research and recent collaborations among scientists who are attempting to identify the composition of all human genetic material have greatly enhanced the ability to detect the genes responsible for many more diseases, including various forms of cancer. Some state laws already require special protection of this information [9].

Protection of patient information that reflects a diagnosis with a **sexually transmitted disease,** such as HIV or AIDS, is clearly required by law because of the social stigma associated with these conditions. Under certain circumstances, some states and the federal government have laws specifically limiting the type and amount of information that can be released from a patient's record. For example, in some states, providers who release information about a patient's **psychological treatment** to a third-party payor, such as a health insurance company, must limit disclosure to administrative information, diagnostic information, patient status, and/or other general information and provide no specific details regarding sessions or other treatment. (Check your specific state laws.)

At the federal level, there are specific standards that limit disclosure of medical records that contain **substance abuse**

Box 9-2 | Sensitive Patient Information

Four types of patient information are entitled to increased protection from inappropriate disclosure because of the sensitive nature of the information:
1. Substance abuse
2. Mental illness
3. Sexually transmitted diseases
4. Genetic makeup

information, such as drug addiction [10]. These are only a few examples of the many state and federal limitations imposed.

■ Measures to Protect the CPR

What are some of the specific measures in place to protect the CPR? Nowadays, each healthcare worker permitted to access the CPR is issued a **confidential personal code (CPC)** or computer password by the employer. The password provides the user with a level of access necessary for the user to perform his or her job. In many states, the regulatory bodies that oversee various healthcare practitioners, such as physicians, have regulations that specifically address access and use of a CPC and the periodic changing of CPCs. An example of such a regulation is set forth in Box 9-3. Most employers strictly prohibit the user from sharing the password with anyone else. In fact, employers will discipline an employee

Box 9-3 | CPR Regulations Example

A patient record may be prepared and maintained on a personal or other computer only when it meets the following criteria:
1. The patient record shall contain ~~at least two forms~~ of identification, for example, name and record number or any other specific information.
2. An entry in the patient record shall be made by the physician contemporaneously with the medical service and shall contain the date of service, date of entry, and full printed name of the treatment provider. The physician shall finalize or "sign" the entry by means of a confidential personal code ("CPC") and include date of the "signing."
3. Alternatively, the physician may dictate a dated entry for later transcription. The transcription shall be dated and identified as "preliminary" until reviewed, finalized, and dated by the responsible physician as provided in (2) above.
4. The system shall contain an internal permanently activated date and time recordation for all entries and shall automatically prepare a backup copy of the file.
5. The system shall be designed in such manner that, after "signing" by means of the CPC, the existing entry cannot be changed in any manner. Notwithstanding the permanent status of a prior entry, a new entry may be made at any time and may indicate correction to a prior entry.
6. Where more than one licensee is authorized to make entries into the computer file of any professional treatment record, the physician responsible for the medical practice shall assure that each such person obtains a CPC and uses the file program in the same manner [11].

who shares the password with others. Disciplinary action may include suspension or possible termination of employment, depending on the facility's policies and the nature of the transgression.

▪ ▪ ▪ What If?

You saw another healthcare provider accessing a patient record using someone else's CPC.
1. What do you do?
2. What are the policies and procedures in your facility regarding accessing a patient's records?

Biometrics

Once the technology becomes more cost effective, more healthcare facilities will begin to utilize **biometrics** in place of passwords to allow healthcare workers access to the CPR. **Biometric identification systems** detect a human physical feature to allow access to computer data. Some examples include fingerprint recognition when an employee touches a special keypad, retina or iris scanning when an employee looks into the computer screen, and voice recognition. This technology will enhance a facility's ability to further restrict inappropriate access to patient information.

Identification

Most CPR systems have the ability to determine the identity of anyone who accesses the system and to detect whether that individual is authorized to do so. CPR systems also have the ability to create audit trails that record all attempts made to access a patient record and all attempts to alter that record. These audit trails also detect and trace a breach in security. All healthcare workers should familiarize themselves with their employer's policies and procedures for reporting suspected security breaches of the computer system.

Protection of Information

For the healthcare worker who uses the computer terminal, whether on a regular basis or intermittently, it is important to protect the information from unauthorized viewers. Computer terminals should be positioned so they cannot be seen by those who have no need to view the information. Computer terminals should also make use of an automatic blanking feature so that the screen will go blank if a keystroke is not made within a set period of time. Too often, healthcare workers also leave computer terminals without signing off—a habit that should be avoided so as to prevent an unauthorized user's access.

▪▪▪ What If?

The medication distribution machine requires your specific identification number to obtain drugs and requires the recording of numbers of those who witness wastage. You are new to the unit and notice a list with everyone's identification numbers taped to the back of the machine.
1. What are the legal implications?
2. What potential problems can arise from this situation?

▪ Handling Requests and Subpoenas for Patient Records

Requests for patient records come from various sources, including the patient, health insurance carriers, managed-care companies, other healthcare providers, and attorneys. All healthcare providers require proper authorization and consent from the patient before such information is released to the requester. Professional groups such as the **Joint Commission on Accreditation of Healthcare Organizations (JCAHO)** mandate such measures. Governmental agencies such as the **Office of the Inspector General (OIG),** which oversees the prevention and investigation of Medicare and Medicaid fraud and abuse, recommend that facilities adopt compliance programs that address, among other things, policies and procedures for the distribution of patient records.

Healthcare facilities frequently receive legal documents, such as a subpoena duces tecum. Attorneys often direct such subpoenas to the patient record custodian, commanding the custodian to appear for a deposition and produce a patient's treatment record. State courts and the federal courts have specific rules addressing the proper form, appropriate service, and other requirements necessary for the subpoena to be valid. (See the Federal Rules of Civil Procedure and your state law regarding the subpoena duces tecum.)

In some states, a subpoena duces tecum must state that the documentation requested shall not be produced or released until the date specified for the taking of the deposition. This provision gives opposing counsel, usually the patient's attorney, the opportunity to quash the subpoena. Opposing counsel may have reason to believe that the subpoenaed information is not at issue in the case, is confidential, and should not be released. If that is the case, a motion to quash the subpoena is filed. It is important that the medical records custodian not release the documentation sought until the date specified in the subpoena. If the medical records custodian receives oral or written notice that opposing counsel has moved to quash the subpoena or is going to do so, the documentation sought should not be released until the facility is provided with a court order.

If any situation arises in which health information personnel are unsure whether to release patient information in response to a subpoena or other request, the patient (or the patient's attorney, if there is one) should be contacted and written authorization obtained.

▪ ▪ ▪ **What If?**

A hospital staff member "obtains" an access code to check on the HIV status of a coworker she is dating.
1. What should you do if you learn of this breach of confidentiality?
2. What are the legal and ethical issues?

Special concerns may be raised if the patient record contains any information that is entitled to increased protection as previously discussed. For example, there may be concerns and uncertainties about releasing medical records containing substance abuse information. Health information personnel should consult the facility's legal counsel before releasing any information if there are concerns or uncertainties as to how to proceed. It is much wiser to exercise caution before the information is released than to attempt to prevent costly litigation after an inappropriate disclosure.

▪ Conclusion

In the case scenario earlier in this chapter, Ester Levin was rightfully concerned about providing Mr. Farmer with a printout of the healthcare records pertaining to Dr. Lewis. All healthcare information should be considered confidential. Although there are certain exceptions to nondisclosure, none of the exceptions applied. Lewis did not authorize release of his records, and Farmer had no need to know what was contained in the healthcare record. In fact, because of possible HIV status, Lewis's record was entitled to heightened protection.

Although Levin was afraid that she might be disciplined or fired if she refused to give Farmer the information he requested, the opposite is true. Had she released the information she would have exposed herself, Farmer, and the medical center to possible litigation. She may have lost her job as a result of her failure to uphold the medical center's policies regarding nondisclosure. The situation called for Levin's firm, but polite, refusal to release the information, accompanied by a brief explanation that her department's policies and procedures do not authorize her to comply with his request.

■ ■ ■ Pertinent Points

1. When in doubt, obtain the patient's consent for release of records.
2. The basic rule of thumb for releasing information is to ask who has a need to know the information contained in the patient's record.
3. Negligence is different from an intentional tort or quasi-intentional tort.
4. Tort is a civil wrongdoing.
5. Breach of confidentiality is a quasi-intentional tort.
6. Sensitive information includes patient information dealing with:
   a. Genetic makeup
   b. Mental illness
   c. Substance abuse
   d. Sexually transmitted disease.
7. *CPC* means "confidential personal code" or computer password.
8. Biometric identification systems are developed as an additional security device to protect the release of patient information.
9. A subpoena duces tecum is used to obtain medical records.
10. Libel is written defamation and slander is oral defamation.

11. Defamation is false communication to a third party that in some way injures the person's reputation, status in the community, and respect held by others.
12. Some patient information is required by state or federal law to be disclosed such as STDs and suspected child or elder abuse.

▪ ▪ ▪ Study Questions

1. What does right to privacy mean with regard to healthcare records?
2. What does the Need-to-Know Exception or rule mean when applied to the release of patient information?
3. Discuss two violations of a patient's right of privacy.
4. Explain how a breach of confidentiality differs from invasion of privacy.
5. What types of patient information are considered sensitive and should receive increased protection?
6. Describe measures that can be used to protect the patient's computerized record.
7. What is a subpoena duces tecum? How is it commonly used with regard to patient records?
8. Describe to the class situations you have been in or have witnessed that could have resulted in litigation due to an invasion of a patient's privacy or a breach of confidentiality. How could the situation have been handled differently?
9. What is a tort?
10. What is a quasi-intentional tort? Give several examples.

▪ ▪ ▪ References

1. Robley v. Blue Cross/Blue Shield of Miss., 935 So.2d 990 (Miss. 2006).
2. Pierce v. Caday, 422 S.E.2d 37 (Va. 1992).
3. Estate of Behringer v. Princeton Med. Ctr. 592 A.2d 1251 (N.J. 1991).
4. Fairfax Hosp. v. Curtis, 492 S.E.2d 642 (Va. 1997).
5. *Id.* at 644.
6. *Id.*
7. Ballard, D. & Cohen, J. W. (1995). Confidentiality of patient records in the computer age. *Journal of Nursing Law,* 2(4), 49–61
8. Proposed Rules, Security and Electronic Signature Standards, 63 Fed. Reg. 43242 (August 12, 1998).
9. Scanlon, C. (1998). The legal implications of genetic testing. *RN,* Mar; 61(3):61–5.
10. 42 U.S.C. § 290(ee-3).
11. N.J.A.C. 13:35–6.5 (3).

■ ■ ■ Resources

Nurse Attorney Institute, LLC, www.NurseLaw.com.

Office for Civil Rights, Department of Health and Human Services, www.hhs.gov/ocr/hipaa.

U.S. government, www.usa.gov.

Clinical Laboratory Liability

Key Chapter Concepts

- Burden of Proof
- Clinical Laboratory Improvement Amendments
- Expert Witness
- Negligence
- Practice Guidelines
- Scope of Duty
- Spoliation
- Standards of Care

Objectives

At the conclusion of this chapter, the reader will be able to:

1. Identify the elements of a professional negligence action.
2. Identify at least five sources of standards of care.
3. Discuss the Clinical Laboratory Improvement Amendments.
4. Define *spoliation*.
5. Explain the expert testimony requirement and exceptions.

■ Introduction

There are many areas of potential legal liability for clinical laboratories, including breach of contract, federal false claims for Medicare and Medicaid billing practices, employer and employee disputes, and negligence. This chapter focuses on areas of potential liability for negligence, also known as malpractice.

> ### Case Scenario
>
> Blood tests are ordered for a patient suffering symptoms of weakness in her lower extremities. The tests are to determine if she has multiple sclerosis or a vitamin B_{12} deficiency. The laboratory incorrectly reports a normal range for vitamin B_{12} as a result of an error in methodology. Vitamin B_{12} tests are ordered again because the patient's symptoms worsen, but the tests are never performed. The patient becomes permanently paralyzed. Who is liable? What breach of the standards occurred? (This case will be discussed later in the chapter.)

■ Negligence

Negligence is the failure to use such care that a reasonably prudent and careful person would use under similar circumstances. It is the act of omission or the commission of an act by a person of ordinary prudence under similar circumstances. What would a person with the same knowledge and experience do under similar circumstances?

There are four elements a claimant, or plaintiff, must prove in a malpractice action:
1. Duty
2. Breach of duty
3. Proximate cause (causal connection)
4. Damages

The plaintiff must prove all four elements by a preponderance of the evidence. In other words, the jury (or a court sitting as the finder of fact) must determine whether in its collective mind, on the basis of the evidence presented, it is more likely than not that the alleged negligence caused injury to the plaintiff. If so, the jury (or court) will determine the amount by which the plaintiff has been damaged.

■ Standard of Care

All persons have a general duty to avoid harming other persons. In the usual negligence case, the "reasonable person" standard is used to determine whether a defendant has breached that duty. In making this determination, the fact finder, jury or judge, must decide whether the defendant acted as an ordinary reasonable person would have acted under the same or similar circumstances. In professional negligence actions, otherwise known as malpractice actions, the professional's conduct is measured by the standards of the profession rather than the reasonable person standard. The professional standards take into account the specialized knowledge, skill, and experience of the professional. Practice guidelines, laws, regulations, or simply the usual day-to-day practices of the members of the profession may embody professional standards. These standards must ordinarily be introduced at a trial through the testimony of an expert witness, as discussed subsequently.

An early procedural issue that courts faced in malpractice litigation was whether the professional standard against which a defendant's conduct was to be measured was determined by looking solely at the usual practices of members of the profession in the same locality as the defendant or by looking at usual practices nationally. At one time, the prevailing rule was that professional conduct was measured against the conduct of other members of the profession who met the minimum qualifications for licensure in the same or similar locale. The majority rule now recognizes a national standard of care with respect to medical specialties and other certified or accredited healthcare services, including clinical laboratories.

The evolution from the local standard and the rationale for a national standard of care in medical negligence cases was directly at issue in *Morrison v. MacNamera* [1].[1] *Morrison* involved a nationally certified clinical laboratory against which a malpractice suit had been filed by a patient injured during the performance of a urethral smear test. The issue on appeal was whether the laboratory, through its employee, had breached the standard of care by performing the test while the patient was standing. There was an additional issue of whether repeating the test with the patient standing when the patient was feeling faint after the first swab was taken was negligent. Expert witnesses testified for the Washington, D.C., laboratory that it was proper to perform the test with the patient in a standing position and that it was the accepted practice in the locality. Experts from other areas of the country testified to the contrary. The court explained the original reason for the locality standard:

---

[1]The court discussed the issue at great length in a comprehensive review of the case law from across the country on the issue, on both local and national standards of care.

This doctrine ... appears to have developed in the late nineteenth century.... The rule was designed to protect doctors in rural areas who, because of inadequate training and experience and lack of effective means of transportation and communication, could not be expected to exhibit the skill and care of urban doctors.... In sum, the locality rule was premised on the notion that the disparity in education and access to advances in medical science between rural and urban doctors required that they be held to different standards of care [2].

After a lengthy dissertation on the subject, the court concluded that the standardization of medical education throughout the country, the availability of medical journals on a nationwide basis, the ubiquitous "detail men" of the drug companies, tape-recorded and closed-circuit television, medical presentations, hundreds of widely available postgraduate courses, and other factors rendered the locality rule obsolete in medical malpractice cases. The court also noted that everyone in a locality following a particular procedure does not make a negligent procedure acceptable. The court held that these same reasons apply with equal validity to hold clinical laboratories to a national standard of care.

■ Clinical Laboratory Improvement Amendments

In *Morrison*, a 1979 case, the laboratory involved was admittedly a nationally certified clinical laboratory. Today, it would be unusual to find a medical laboratory that is not certified, accredited, or otherwise subject to national regulatory standards. In 1988, Congress passed the Clinical Laboratory Improvement Amendments (CLIA) [3].[2] Through the CLIA, the Centers for Medicare and Medicaid regulate all laboratory testing (except research) performed on humans in the United States. The CLIA Program, implemented by the Division of Laboratory Services under the Medicaid and State Operations (CMSO), has the primary goal of ensuring quality laboratory testing. CLIA has no direct Medicare or Medicaid program responsibilities, although all clinical labs must be properly certified to receive payments from Medicare or Medicaid. The CLIA set

---

[2]It should be noted that as of December 2006, the states of Washington and New York were exempt from CLIA regulations (www.cms.hhs.gov/clia).

forth extensive conditions or standards that laboratories[3] must meet to receive certification from the U.S. Department of Health and Human Services (HHS).[4] Unless a clinical laboratory performs only simple, routine tests for which CLIA has waived certification,[5] a laboratory must be certified by HHS or another approved accrediting organization to receive payments for services to Medicare or Medicaid beneficiaries. CLIA regulations include standards for proficiency testing by specialty and subspecialty, quality control, quality assurance, personnel qualifications and responsibilities, facilities, equipment, and test-specific procedures (Box 10-1). The significance of the regulations to potential malpractice liability is that the comprehensive regulations set a minimum standard against which the conduct of a laboratory or its personnel will be undoubtedly measured in litigation.[6] These standards can be introduced at trial through the testimony of an expert witness as evidence of the laboratory's breach of duty of care to its clients. If the failure of the laboratory to meet regulatory standards causes injury to a patient, malpractice liability will be difficult to avoid.[7]

---

[3]Laboratory is defined as "a facility for the biological, microbiological, serological, chemical, immunohematological, hematological, biophysical, cytological, pathological, or other examination of materials derived from the human body for the purpose of providing information for the diagnosis, prevention, or treatment of any disease or impairment of, or the assessment of the health of human beings" 42 C.F.R. § 493.2.

[4]The regulations implementing CLIA are codified at 42 C.F.R. § 493.

[5]A list of waived tests is set forth in the regulations at 42 C.F.R. § 493.15.

[6]The unexcused violation of a statute or regulation enacted for the safety of the public that is applicable under the circumstances is per se or automatic negligence in some states. This rule is known as "negligence per se," and proof of "violation" of the safety statute or regulation establishes the breach of duty.

[7]Although the overall burden of proof on a plaintiff in a negligence action is "preponderance of the evidence" or "more likely than not," an expert's testimony with respect to the cause of the plaintiff's injury must meet a more stringent standard in most jurisdictions. The expert must testify that the breach of the standard of care probably, not possibly, caused the injury (e.g., *Denneny v. Siegal*, 407 F.2d 433, 400–41 (3rd Cir. 1969).

Box 10-1 | CLIA Quality Control for Tests of Moderate Complexity, High Complexity, or Any Combination of Tests

The Code of Federal Regulations includes standards and conditions for the following [4]:

493.1203 Standard: Moderate- or high-complexity testing, or both, effective December 31, 2000

493.1204 Standard: Facilities

493.1204 Standard: Test methods, equipment, instrumentation, reagents, materials, and supplies

493.1211 Standard: Procedure manual

493.1213 Standard: Establishment and verification of method performance

493.1215 Standard: Equipment maintenance and function checks

493.1217 Standard: Calibration and calibration verification procedures

493.1218 Standard: Control procedures

493.1219 Standard: Remedial actions

493.1221 Standard: Quality-control records

493.1223 Standard: Condition: Quality control—specialties and subspecialties for tests of moderate and high complexity

493.1225 Condition: Microbiology

493.1227 Condition: Bacteriology

493.1229 Condition: Microbacteriology

493.1231 Condition: Mycology

493.1233 Condition: Parasitology

493.1235 Condition: Virology

493.1237 Condition: Diagnostic immunology

493.1239 Condition: Syphilis serology

493.1241 Condition: General immunology

493.1243 Condition: Chemistry

493.1245 Condition: Routine chemistry

493.1247 Condition: Endocrinology

493.1249 Condition: Toxicology

493.1251 Condition: Urinalysis

493.1255 Condition: Pathology

493.1259 Condition: Histopathology

493.1261 Condition: Oral pathology

493.1263 Condition: Radiobioassay

493.1265 Condition: Histocompatibility

493.1267 Condition: Clinical cytogenics

493.1269 Condition: Immunohematology

493.1271 Condition: Transfusion services and blood banking

493.1273 Standard: Immunohematological collection, processing, dating periods, labeling, and distribution of blood and blood products

493.1275 Standard: Blood and blood-product storage facilities

493.1277 Standard: Arrangement for services

493.1283 Standard: Provision of testing

493.1283 Standard: Retention of samples of transfused blood

493.1285 Standard: Investigation of transfusion reactions

─────────────────────────── ■ ■ ■ **What If?**

Your friend was called to do a random drug screen and, because you work in the lab, she asked you to "give her a sample" because she used illegal drugs at a party last night and does not want to get fired. What should you do? What are the legal and ethical implications?

■ Sources of Standards

Additional federal regulations apply to clinical laboratories located in hospital facilities. The Conditions of Participation for Hospitals for Laboratory Services [5] specifically incorporate all CLIA standards and make them applicable to hospital facilities. Other regulations applicable to hospital laboratories are included, which are principally directed toward handling of potentially infected blood and blood products. Professional organizations also promulgate standards and guidelines that may be introduced at trial to establish a duty and prove breach of that duty in a laboratory malpractice action. The American Board of Clinical Chemistry offers certification in clinical chemistry, toxicological chemistry, and molecular diagnostics to individuals with doctoral-level degrees.[8] The board also establishes standards of competence for those who practice clinical laboratory medicine (www.aacc.org/abcc/). The American Association for Clinical Chemistry maintains a list of standard materials and standard methods compiling the most up-to-date information on clinical laboratory standardization available to its Standards Committee.[9] The National Academy of Clinical Biochemistry publishes "Laboratory Medicine Practice Guidelines" (LMPG) for the application of clinical biochemistry to medical diagnosis and therapy. Standards may also be established by a laboratory's own internal policies and procedures manuals.

─────────────────────────── ■ ■ ■ **What If?**

You find a missing lab result that is abnormal. The patient has died and the cause pertains to the abnormal results. What do you do? What are the legal and ethical issues?

───────────────────────────

[8]ABCC, 1850 K Street, NW, Suite 625, Washington, DC 20006-2213 (phone: 202-835-8727; Fax 202-833-4576).
[9]Same address as note 8. Standards are available on line at www.aacc.org.

■ Expert Witness

Expert witnesses are generally required to establish the applicable standard of care in laboratory malpractice actions, as they do in other medical malpractice cases. The testimony of an expert in clinical laboratory science or other related disciplines is necessary to explain the technical and scientific data that a lay jury need to identify the appropriate standard of care and to determine whether that standard has been breached.[10] An exception to the expert testimony requirement, known as the "common knowledge" exception, was at issue in *Schindel v. Albany Medical Corporation* [6]. This exception applies where "the defendant's negligence is so grossly apparent or the treatment is so common that a lay person can readily appraise it using his everyday knowledge" [7].

In *Schindel*, a woman sought an abortion at a local women's clinic. The laboratory analysis of the tissue following the procedure indicated the possibility of an ectopic pregnancy that the abortion procedure did not terminate. The testimony at trial established that although the physician had a duty to review the laboratory report to identify any abnormal results, it was the duty of the laboratory personnel to notify the patient of the findings and to give her instructions. In *Schindel*, alleged efforts to notify the plaintiff by mail and telephone were unsuccessful, the plaintiff did not receive notice, and the ectopic pregnancy ruptured. The plaintiff alleged that the defendant was negligent in failing to employ and enforce proper procedures to notify her of the abnormal laboratory findings and failed to notify her of the possible ectopic pregnancy. Without expert testimony to establish the standard of care, the jury returned a verdict for the plaintiff.

On appeal, the laboratory successfully argued that the verdict should be reversed owing to the lack of expert testimony. The court found that the common knowledge exception did not apply to the case even though neither the quality of treatment nor the correctness of the physician's diagnosis was at issue.

---

[10]An individual may qualify to testify as an expert in litigation on the basis of his or her knowledge, skill, experience, training, or education in the field. It is the function of the trial judge as a "gatekeeper" to determine whether an individual qualifies to testify as an expert. Fed. R. Evid. 702; *United States v. Webb*, 115 F.3d 711 (9th Cir. 1997); *Wood v. Minnesota Mining and Mfg. Co.*, 112 F.3d 306, 309 (8th Cir. 1997); *Bogosian v. Mercedes-Benz*, 104 F.3d 472, 476 (1st Cir. 1997).

The court concluded that it was the "urgency of the danger involved and the likelihood and extent of harm to the plaintiff which would dictate the extent of the defendant's duty to notify the plaintiff" [8] and these factors required expert testimony.

■ Scope of Duty

Another aspect of the legal concept of duty in a malpractice case is whether a duty to a particular individual exists under the circumstances. In the physician-patient context, a physician's duty to provide medical care that meets accepted minimum standards begins at the inception of the physician-patient relationship. As in the physician context, the contours and scope of a laboratory's duty of care are not always a bright line. In a Wyoming Supreme Court case [9], the question was whether a specimen collection company owed a duty to an employee of the employer, which had hired the company to collect urine specimens for drug and alcohol screening. The court held that there was a duty, thus overruling the lower court. To collect urine specimens from randomly selected employees, the employer had retained the collection company. The collection company contracted with another laboratory to analyze the specimens and to report the results. The plaintiff was randomly selected for testing, gave a specimen in an unsealed container, and then returned to the restroom to wash his hands. In his absence, the container was sealed and the plaintiff was directed to initial the label. Plaintiff's employer was subsequently notified that the laboratory results demonstrated a 0.32 urine alcohol content, which indicated the plaintiff was grossly drunk at the time of his testing, 10 hours into his shift. On the basis of this report, the plaintiff was terminated from his employment. The plaintiff filed suit against the collection company alleging that the employee who collected the specimen:
1. Was inadequately trained;
2. Failed to employ proper procedures;
3. Failed to inform the plaintiff that specific urinalysis procedures were not followed; and
4. Misrepresented to the plaintiff the accuracy and reliability of urine alcohol testing.

The court explained that a duty exists where, "upon the facts in evidence, such a relation exists between the parties that the community will impose a legal obligation upon one for the benefit of the other—or more simply, whether the interest of the plaintiff which has suffered invasion was entitled to legal protection at the hands of the defendant" [10]. The court noted that other courts were in disagreement with its opinion on the issue.[11]

Determination of the existence of a duty, according to the Wyoming Supreme Court, requires balancing of the following:

1. The foreseeability of harm to the plaintiff;
2. The closeness of the connection between the defendant's conduct and the injury suffered;
3. The degree of certainty that the plaintiff suffered injury;
4. The moral blame attached to the defendant's conduct;
5. The policy of preventing future harm;
6. The extent of the burden on the defendant;
7. The consequences to the community and the court system; and
8. The availability, cost, and prevalence of insurance for the risk involved.

In the recent case *Santos v. Kim* [11], the court discussed at length the existence of a duty owed by the director of a medical laboratory to the plaintiff mother of a deceased newborn. The question was whether the director was potentially liable for the laboratory's failure to have policies and procedures in place to ensure that treating physicians were promptly notified of abnormal test results. The court noted that in modern medical practice, it was not always necessary that there be a personal relationship or actual physical contact between the healthcare provider and patient because, in many instances, it is the technician with the least knowledge and skill who actually interacts directly with the patient, as often occurs in radiology and laboratory services. The plaintiff was Rh-negative, and this was her second pregnancy. Her obstetricians had been monitoring her anti-D titers on a biweekly basis to ensure prompt treatment of Rh incompatibility, if necessary. The week the titers rose substantially, the obstetricians were not notified of the abnormal result for two weeks. In the meantime, plaintiff underwent a Cesarean section without prophylactic treatment, which allegedly led to the death of the newborn. The Massachusetts Supreme Court held that under this set of circumstances, the medical director of the laboratory could

---

[11]*See Smith Kline Beecham Corp. v. Doe,* 903 S.W.2d 347 (Tex. 1995), and *Willis v. Roche Biomedical Labs, Inc.,* 61 F.3d 313, 316 (5th Cir. 1995) (finding that a drug tester retained by an employer to screen potential employees owes no duty to that potential employee); *see also Caputo v. Compuchem Labs.,* Civ. A. No. 92-6123, 1994 WL 100084 (E.D. Pa. Feb. 23, 1994), and *Herbert v. Placid Ref. Co.,* 564 So. 2d 371, 374 (La.), *writ denied,* 569 So. 2d 981 (La. 1990).

potentially be liable to the plaintiff even though he had no direct contact with her at any time.

■ Common Areas of Laboratory Liability

Common sources of professional liability (Box 10-2) for clinical laboratories based on reported malpractice cases include the following:
- Error in diagnostic testing for cancer
- False-positive drug screening reported to employers
- Unidentified tainted blood products
- Failure to identify genetic disorders in newborns and pregnancy screening
- Delay in or failure to transmit laboratory results
- Use of improper equipment or procedures

In *Paulk,* plaintiff had a mole removed that was diagnosed as a benign lesion [12]. Four years later, the plaintiff was admitted and diagnosed as suffering from a metastatic cancerous lesion to his brain caused by metastatic malignant melanoma. The original specimen was reexamined, and it was concluded that it was not benign but a primary nodular malignant melanoma. The plaintiff died approximately three months later. The claim is that the pathologists negligently failed to correctly diagnose and report the malignancy in 1991 and that CLA (pathology laboratory) was negligent under the theory of respondeat superior. Defendants admit that the diagnosis was incorrect but that it did not have a causal relationship to the death of the patient. They alleged the melanoma had already metastasized into the blood vessels beyond the skin and that no treatment could have prolonged his life.

Box 10-2 | Common Areas of Laboratory Liability

- Errors in diagnostic testing for cancer
- Errors in reading Pap smears
- False-positive drug screening reported to employers
- Unidentified tainted blood products
- Failure to identify genetic disorders in newborns and pregnancy screening
- Delay in or failure to transmit laboratory results
- Use of improper equipment or procedures

Plaintiff moved for a mistrial and a new trial on the grounds that the expert's testimony (regarding the melanoma cells in the blood vessels) was not disclosed in discovery and resulted in unfair and prejudicial surprise and deprived plaintiff of a fair trial. The court reversed and remanded the case for a new trial.

▪▪▪ What If?

Your coworker is performing a drug screen on someone you intensely dislike. You see she accidentally mixes up the urine specimens and labels them with the wrong name.
What should you do?
What are the legal and ethical implications?

In most reported court cases, whether the defendant's conduct was negligent is not the issue before the court. The court opinions discuss various procedural questions in the context of the malpractice action in which the inappropriateness of the conduct is not questioned. (Most cases that do not have unresolved legal issues to be decided are ultimately settled by the parties and not reported in the case law.)

Pathology errors are very common sources of malpractice liability for clinical laboratories, with allegedly misread Pap smears heading the list. In none of the cases reviewed was the negligence of the conduct even discussed. In *Calvin v. Schlossman* [13], the issue was whether an action alleging that the laboratory was culpable for an error in reading a Pap smear is subject to state law prelitigation hearing procedures applicable to medical malpractice actions. The court held that it was. In *Riseman v. Goldberg* [14], the court questioned whether the private physician who ordered a test or the hospital, which operated the laboratory that was vicariously responsible for the pathologist's error in reading a Pap smear specimen, was culpable.[12] In *Berg v. Footer* [15], liability to the plaintiff was stipulated. The only question was whether the settling defendant was a "joint tortfeasor" for purposes of determining the allowable deduction from the judgment owed plaintiff by the nonsettling defendant. *Bergherr v. Sommer* [16] discusses whether a Minnesota court has jurisdiction over an out-of-state laboratory in which a Minnesota laboratory off-loaded specimens. The court ruled that it had jurisdiction because the out-of-state laboratory

---

[12]Vicarious liability is defined as indirect legal responsibility, such as the liability of an employer for the acts of an employee, or of a principal for the torts and contracts of an agent.

actively solicited business from Minnesota through its agreements with the Minnesota laboratory and benefited economically from "voluntary interstate economic activity" [17].

Marsh v. Wentzel [18] deals with the statute of limitations for misdiagnosed breast cancer that was not discovered until after the four-year time limit for bringing suit had expired. *Henry v. Metropolitan Government of Nashville* [19] points out that even though there may be negligent conduct, if the negligence does not cause any damage, there is no basis to recover in a malpractice lawsuit and the case will be dismissed. In *Henry*, plaintiff had a Pap smear in July 1993 that tested positive for cervical cancer, but she was never informed of the results. In October 1994, she had another Pap smear that was reported to her as positive, and as a result she had surgery. The testimony of experts established that although there was a 14-month delay in notifying her of the cervical cancer, there was no damage because she underwent the same surgery she would have had earlier had the diagnosis been made earlier. Accordingly, there was no harm suffered and the case was dismissed.

Equipment and procedural errors are often the subject of laboratory liability cases. In *National Health Laboratories v. Pari* [20], the example given in the case scenario, an error in testing methodology resulted in a $10 million verdict for a patient permanently paralyzed owing to an error in diagnosis. Blood tests were ordered for the plaintiff, who was suffering symptoms of weakness in her lower extremities, to differentiate between multiple sclerosis and vitamin B_{12} deficiency. The laboratory admitted the error in methodology, which had caused the technicians to incorrectly reach a normal-range finding for vitamin B_{12}. When the symptoms worsened, the patient was admitted to the hospital and vitamin B_{12} tests were again ordered, but this time the order was never carried out. The laboratory and the hospital were both held to be 50% responsible for the plaintiff's resulting paralysis and damages.

─── ▪ ▪ ▪ **What If?**

You see a senior coworker using antiquated equipment and methods.
What do you do?
How can this affect patient care?
What are the legal and ethical implications?

AIDS- and hepatitis-tainted blood products were areas of significant liability for laboratories and hospitals in the early 1980s, even in the absence of negligence, before AIDS was identified and a reliable test existed to screen blood products for HIV contamination. Many states now have statutes that preclude strict liability or liability without fault in these cases, although liability for negligent screening still exists. (Check your state's statutes).

In *Smith v. County of Kern* [21], a laboratory performed the wrong test on a blood sample. An HIV test was ordered pursuant to state law for the benefit of a police officer exposed to the blood of a patient who said he tried to commit suicide because he suffered from AIDS. The blood sample given by the patient was erroneously tested for hepatitis instead of the HIV virus, but the remaining sample was discarded before the error was discovered. The patient had also been discharged, leaving no forwarding address by this time. It took more than six months to locate the patient to obtain another sample and perform the proper tests. The court agreed there was possible liability for the six-month delay in obtaining results of the HIV test.

While spoliation was not an issue in the *Smith* case, the spoliation doctrine has been developing over the past decade as both an evidentiary rule and a source of punishment or sanctions against defendants and their attorneys who lose or destroy evidence or alter records. **Spoliation** is defined as the intentional destruction of evidence that, when established, enables the court to instruct the jury that it may infer that the lost or damaged evidence was unfavorable to the party responsible for the spoliation. It includes "the destruction or the significant and meaningful alteration of a document or instrument." In *Aldrich v. Roche Biomedical Laboratories, Inc.* [22], the court concluded there was no spoliation because it could not be definitively determined how pathology slides disappeared or who was at fault. The pathology slides that were questionably misread disappeared in the court or after being returned by mail from an expert reviewing the slides for a second opinion. The loss of the slides was ultimately determined not to affect the presentation of the case.

The CLIA contains specific requirements for record keeping and preservation of samples. Records of patient testing, including printed results, immunohematology records, transfusion records, and records of blood and blood-product testing must be retained. (Check the CLIA Web site for the most recent requirements.) A laboratory has an affirmative duty not only to not lose, alter, or destroy records but also to maintain them.

―――――――――――――――――――――――**▪ ▪ ▪ What If?**

You see a coworker slip pathology slides into his pocket that are at issue and evidence in a malpractice case.
What do you do?
What are the legal implications?

▪ Conclusion

As in other areas of healthcare liability, theories of liability evolve as professional standards change. It is incumbent on the practitioner to constantly stay abreast of new standards and regulations, to be familiar with and follow in-house policies and procedures, and to question out-of-date practices, equipment, and methodologies (Box 10-3).

Box 10-3 | Clinical Laboratories Improvement Amendments (CLIA)

- Congress passed CLIA in 1988 to establish quality standards for all non-research laboratory testing performed on human specimens for the purpose of providing information for diagnosis, treatment, prevention, or health assessment.
- Laboratories are required to be certified by the Secretary of the Department of Health and Human Services (DHHS).
- CLIA standards are national and apply to all providers rendering clinical laboratory services.

▪ ▪ ▪ Study Questions

1. What are the elements of negligence?
2. List four areas of potential legal liability for clinical laboratories.
3. Discuss local versus national standards of care. How do they differ?
4. Find a case in your field at the law library or online and discuss the elements of negligence.
5. What are the Clinical Laboratory Improvement Amendments?
6. List three sources of standards for your area of practice.
7. List six common areas of laboratory liability and how to prevent lawsuits in each area.
8. Find and discuss a case in the following areas:
   a. Pathology error
   b. Misdiagnosed cancer

     c. Equipment error

     d. Procedural error

     e. AIDS-tainted blood products

     f. Hepatitis-tainted blood products.

9. What is spoliation of evidence?
10. What is the burden of proof for a plaintiff in a negligence action?
11. Find standards of care applicable to your area of practice and share with the class.
12. Find a recent case in your state and discuss the breaches of the standard of care and findings of the court.
13. Discuss the duties of an expert witness.
14. Find a resource applicable to your area of practice and share with your class.

■ ■ ■ References

1. Morrison v. MacNamera, 407 A.2d 555 (D.C. 1979).
2. Schindel v. Albany Med. Corp., 252 Ill. App. 3d 389, 395, 625 N.E.2d 114, 119 (1993).
3. Clinical Laboratory Improvement Amendment, Pub. L. No. 100–578.
4. 42 C.F.R § 493(k). www.archives.gov.
5. Conditions of Participation for Hospitals for Laboratory Services, 42 C.F.R. § 482.27.
6. Schindel v. Albany Med. Corp., 625 N.E.2d 114, (Ill. 1993).
7. *Id.* at 119.
8. *Id.*
9. Duncan v. Afton, Inc., 991 P.2d 739 (Wyo. 1999).
10. *Id.* at 32.
11. Santos v. Kim, 706 N.E.2d 658 (Mass. 1999).
12. Paulk v. Cent. Lab. Assocs., 636 N.W.2d 170 (Neb. 2001).
13. Calvin v. Schlossman, 74 A.D. 265 (N.Y. 1980).
14. Riseman v. Goldberg, 581 N.Y.S.2d 854 (N.Y. 1992).
15. Berg v. Footer, 673 A.2d 1244 (D.C. 03/22/1996).
16. Bergherr v. Sommer, 523 N.W.2d 17 (Minn. 1994).
17. *Id.* at 52.
18. Marsh v. Wentzel, 732 So. 2d 985 (Ala. 1998).
19. Henry v. Metro. Gov't of Nashville, App. Lexis at *303 (Tenn. 1999).
20. Nat'l Health Labs. v. Pari, 596 A.2d 555 (D.C. 1991).
21. Smith v. County of Kern, 20 Cal. App. 4th 1826 (Cal. 1993).
22. Aldrich v. Roche Biomedical Labs., Inc., 737 So. 2d 1124 (Fla. 1999).

■ ■ ■ Resources

Nurse Attorney Institute, www.nurselaw.com.

11

Medical Equipment Liability and Litigation

Key Chapter Concepts

- Code of Ethics
- Liability
- Medical Device
- Product Liability
- Safe Medical Devices Act of 1990
- Sentinel Event
- Strict Liability

Objectives

At the conclusion of this chapter, the reader will be able to:

1. Define the liability that arises in professions when using medical equipment.
2. Identify potential and/or actual medical equipment litigation.
3. Discuss the Safe Medical Devices Act.
4. Discuss common areas of liability for licensed professionals.
5. Identify strategies for reducing and/or eliminating liability.

■ Introduction

The focus of this chapter is on common areas of liability and litigation associated with medical equipment. The chapter provides information related to medical equipment liability and litigation, examples of medical equipment liability and litigation, and strategies for reducing and/or eliminating liability associated with the use of medical equipment.

Case Scenario

In an effort to alleviate a stricture, a patient had a Foley catheter inserted during surgery. Several days later, healthcare providers discovered a tiny hole in the balloon of the catheter that allowed urine to leak through to the suture line and into the tissue. This situation caused the patient to undergo two additional surgeries. Who was found negligent? Why? What would you do if you are named in a lawsuit for being negligent in providing safe care to a client? You pride yourself as being a competent and knowledgeable professional. As you investigate the situation, you learn that the negligence is related to a malfunctioning piece of equipment. You are puzzled because you reported that piece of faulty equipment to your supervisor. What can you do? What should you have done? How could you have prevented the injury to the patient? What documentation do you need to protect yourself?

Liability is an individual's responsibility for his or her conduct for failure to meet a standard of care or for failure to perform a duty that causes harm to a client [1, 2]. **Strict liability** differs in that liability may be proved without demonstrating fault. **Product liability** is the liability of a manufacturer or vendor for injury to a person by a given product [3].

Is the issue of liability the equipment or the operator? What do you think as you read the following?

• A burn is caused from a heating pad placed on a shivering infant [4].
• A patient is left without oxygen for a period of time while a caregiver looks for a portable tank [5].
• A medication burn occurs to a patient's chest-wall incision from Nipride leaking through a pinhole in an atrial catheter during surgery [6].
• Equipment is substituted because the right equipment is not available [7].

■ The Safe Medical Device Act of 1990

What constitutes a medical device or medical equipment? *Medical device* is a broad term encompassing such items as implants, single-use disposable devices, instruments, machines, apparatus, and reagents. The **Safe Medical Devices Act of 1990 (SMDA)** provides rules and regulations for the safety and reporting of medical devices. Under the SMDA, healthcare facilities must report serious or potentially serious device-related injuries or illnesses of patients and/or employees to the device's manufacturer [8]. If death from a device has occurred, it must be reported to the **Food and Drug Administration (FDA)**. Healthcare workers and hospitals must also track and report certain information regarding FDA-specified devices upon receipt, removal, or implantation of the device. Devices that must be reported include but are not limited to sutures, heart valves, pacemakers, wheelchairs, gurneys, catheters, infusion pumps, dialysis machines, sponges, and artificial valves or joints. Failure to comply results in civil penalties [9].

Sentinel events are unexpected occurrences of death or serious physical or psychological injury. Sentinel events are voluntarily reported to the Joint Commission on the Accreditation of Healthcare Organizations. The goals of reporting are to continuously improve the quality and safety of health care.

As technology advances and health care becomes more complex, liability risks may increase. The risks do not increase for any one organization; individuals assume equal risk and professional responsibility to ensure their knowledge of and competency in those advances. Medical equipment has incorporated the use of computerization or information systems technology. For many individuals who are still not comfortable with computerization, such technology poses a new challenge. Healthcare professionals and organizations can safeguard against potential liability by identifying the need for knowledge and education, assuming responsibility for obtaining that education, and ensuring competency through mentorship and certifications.

Registered nurses and licensed allied healthcare professionals (e.g., physical therapists, occupational therapists, respiratory therapists) take an oath to safeguard the client with competent and responsible actions. Professional associations have established codes of ethics to uphold the **standards of practice.** Although each profession is unique, many of the standards are similar [9–13]:

- Respecting human dignity
- Safeguarding the client's right to privacy and maintaining confidentiality
- Providing safe and competent care to clients
- Maintaining professional competence and participating in activities to further develop one's education and body of knowledge
- Safeguarding the client/public from misinformation
- Collaborating with other healthcare professionals to promote efforts to meet the needs of the community or client

▪▪▪ What If?

A thermal pad burns a patient. The nursing assistant hides the pad and throws it away. You find the discarded thermal pad. What should you do? What are the legal and ethical implications?

■ Who Is Liable in Equipment Cases?

Cases of malpractice and negligence revolve around practice issues such as errors in medication, treatment, and surgery. The number of medical equipment liability lawsuits continues to grow, especially in the era of advanced technology and the increased use of healthcare devices and equipment. Injury from a device or medical equipment may involve a primary caregiver, organization, and/or equipment manufacturer [11].

Negligence theory or product liability law may be applied to medical equipment liability. Product liability is different from malpractice in that the patient may not have to prove a deviation from a standard of care if the courts apply a strict liability standard. With a strict liability standard, the equipment's manufacturer may be held liable. However, manufacturers may defend themselves by claiming that the negligence was "user error" [12] (Case Example 11-1).

Case Example 11-1

A patient is on intravenous (IV) Heparin at an ordered rate of 10 ml per hour. Upon checking the IV, a nurse discovers the pump is set for 110 ml per hour, 11 times the prescribed dose. The patient's clotting time is at a potentially dangerous level. The patient dies [13]. Certainly, this is a gross medication error. Is this a medical equipment error as well? No, the error that occurred was a "user error" of the equipment.

■ Medication Administration

According to an **Institute of Medicine** report, medical errors are the eighth-leading cause of death in the United States and may be responsible for approximately 98,000 deaths annually. Medication errors are the most common medical errors and the leading causes of injury to patients and of malpractice suits [14]. Is medication administration competency really any different from user or operator competency? Medication administration requires knowledge of the medication, indication, side effects, adverse reactions, dosage, administration, and outcome. It is a professional's responsibility to know and understand medication before administering a medication. Medical equipment requires knowledge of the equipment, indication for use, troubleshooting, resource management, and outcome.

▪ ▪ ▪ What If?

You enter a patient's room and find that the alarm is turned off. You ask the nurse in charge and she tells you to leave it off because it is sounding too often and is "irritating." What do you do? What are the potential legal and ethical problems? Is this malpractice? Is this providing proper care? Are there disciplinary actions that could result because of a patient safety issue? What are the potential dangers to the patient?

▪ Common Types of Errors

Most errors or liabilities occur from lack of knowledge, failure to communicate, failure to follow through, failure to document, misuse, and carelessness [15] (Box 11-1). In the case of a five-month-old boy who was shivering postoperatively, a heating pad was placed on the infant to warm him. The infant sustained second- and third-degree burns to his buttocks [16]. In the case of transferring a patient to a new room, the oxygen-flow meter did not secure in the outlet; the caregiver proceeded to look for an oxygen tank and left the patient without oxygen. The patient went into respiratory arrest and died.

Box 11-1 | Causes of Liability

1. Lack of knowledge
2. Failure to communicate
3. Failure to follow through
4. Failure to document
5. Misuse
6. Carelessness

Equipment that is malfunctioning must be taken out of service. Also, continued assessment and evaluation of patient care is necessary to ensure the meeting of standards of care.

■ Strategies for Reducing or Eliminating Liabilities

There are many articles published on perioperative nursing and electrosurgical safety and other safety measures in the perioperative setting. A committee of the Association of Perioperative Registered Nurses (AORN) has developed recommended practice strategies that include in part the following:

1. Products are to be safe, meet the needs identified, and promote quality patient care.
2. Equipment should be designed to minimize risks of alternate site injuries, capacitive coupling injuries, unintentional activation, and stray currents that can injure patients.
3. A mechanism for evaluation and standardization of medical equipment should be implemented.
4. Evaluation of products should be based on objective criteria specific to the function and use of the device.
5. Safety and warning alarms should be operational at all times.
6. A trial evaluation should be conducted and analyzed.
7. Written policies and procedures must be readily available.

Other strategies to reduce and/or eliminate medical equipment liability and litigation include the following:

- *Increase in knowledge of the equipment:* learn its purpose and indication for use.
- *User competency:* obtain training specific to the equipment and troubleshooting strategies.
- *Communication:* maintain clear and concise communication with all personnel.
- *Follow through:* ensure that faulty equipment is taken out of service and labeled, document out of service, and obtain working equipment for the patient's needs.
- *Documentation:* ensure that proper documentation is reflected in the medical record; concerns may be documented on a quality report; medical equipment failure should be reported according to rules and regulations and sent to appropriate departments for service and repair. (In product liability cases, the maintenance records for the equipment in question may be requested or subpoenaed; see AORN's Recommended Practices for all recommendations at **www.aorn.org**.)
- *Misuse and/or carelessness:* address with colleagues and with management team.

■ Minimize Risks

For all licensed healthcare professionals, practice must continuously be monitored. Individual responsibility for continuing education and keeping up to date is of the utmost importance. Areas in which healthcare professionals must invest their time include new technologies, new treatment modalities, equipment advances, medications, and policies and procedures (Box 11-2). Healthcare professionals must also be familiar with their respective code of ethics, professional standards, and accreditation standards.

Competence is the ability to provide a level of care according to a standard of care and according to the profession's code of ethics. **Incompetence** is the failing of moral commitment in upholding the code of ethics. Incompetence jeopardizes patient safety and

Box 11-2 | Common Medical Equipment That Healthcare Professionals May Encounter

Nursing Assistants/Medical Assistants

- Blood pressure monitors
- Cardiac monitors
- Heart catheters
- Foley catheters
- Heat lamps
- Wheelchairs
- Compression stockings
- Chest tubes
- Gomco

Respiratory

- Ventilators
- Oxygen-flow meters
- Respiratory treatments
- Pulse oximetry
- Compressed-air meters
- Pulmonary function

Physical Therapy

- Whirlpools
- Exercise equipment
- Ambulation belts
- Walkers and canes

Continued

Box 11-2 | Common Medical Equipment That Healthcare Professionals May Encounter—cont'd

- PulseVac system
- Continuous positive motion (CPM) machine

Dental Assistants/Hygienists

- X-ray machine
- Ultrasonic scaler/sonic scaler
- Airbrasive unit
- Air polisher
- Slow-speed hand piece/high-speed hand piece
- Dental unit
- Ultrasonic unit
- Autoclave/chemclave machine
- X-ray developer
- Automated periodontal probe
- Computer, chairside and front office
- Intraoral camera
- Amalgam titrator
- Curing light
- Model trimmer
- Stone or plaster
- Vacuum former
- Power mixing machine
- Lathe
- Panorex machine
- Pulp vitality tester
- Nitrous oxide unit
- Automated irrigating syringe
- Electrocautery machine
- Apex locator
- Casting machine

Occupational Therapy

- Stoves
- Washing machines
- Games

Nursing

- Electronic thermometers
- Blood pressure cuff with sphygmomanometer
- Stethoscope
- Intravenous pumps
- Emerson or Gomco units
- Tube-feeding pumps

- Aqua heating pads (e.g., K pads)
- Hypothermia unit
- Telemetry transmitters and monitors
- Bedside electrocardiogram monitors
- Balloon pumps
- Cardiac monitor and defibrillator
- Specialty beds (e.g., low air loss, rotation, fluidized air)
- Wheelchair stretchers
- Walkers
- Blood glucose meters
- Automatic external defibrillator

Cardiology

- Electrocardiographic unit and leads
- Treadmill
- Cardiac ultrasound unit
- ECG or EKG

Laboratory

- Hematology and chemistry equipment

Perioperative Services (SDS/OR/PACU)

- Electrocautery unit
- Operating room tables
- Operating room instruments
- Anesthesia machine that includes oxygen and nitrous oxide sources

Radiology

- General X-ray or radiographic unit, stationary or mobile
- Fluoroscopy unit
- Nuclear medicine unit
- Magnetic resonance imaging
- Computed tomography
- Digital radiography
- Mammography
- Lithotripters
- Laser
- Angiography or cardiac catheterization equipment
- Lead apron
- Stretchers

Ultrasound

- Doppler
- Unit
- Scanners
- Transducers

well-being. Furthermore, colleagues are placed at risk when they are unable to depend on a team member.

Why does incompetence occur? Apathy, inability to do the work, disorganization, lack of knowledge of necessary pathophysiology, lack of manual dexterity, and irresponsibility are several reasons. Incompetence is generally easily recognizable, but it is still allowed and tolerated. The author Haddad [17] points out three reasons that incompetence is tolerated:

1. Loyalty to colleagues: people make allowances for a person's shortcomings based on their trusting nature.
2. Principle of beneficence: do good for others.
3. The ability of the incompetent professional to manipulate colleagues: place blame.

Competence equals professionalism; therefore, incompetence cannot be tolerated. It is the responsibility of all professionals to maintain standards and to report any deviation in those standards. Loyalty and beneficence cannot be allowed to blur reality. Patient and colleague safety is at stake.

Continued competency is now required in most states and for most professions. Various mechanisms are used to determine continued competency, such as self-evaluations, continuing education programs, and peer review. Most state boards require mandatory continuing education. The cost associated with continuing education is nominal compared to the risks involved in "keeping up" with new trends, techniques, and information in your profession. Investment in training and continuing education minimizes the areas of clinical negligence [18].

▪▪▪ What If?

You see a nursing assistant with a faulty blood pressure cuff that gives incorrect readings. You tell her to get a new one and she ignores you. What are the legal and ethical implications? What should you do?

▪ Conclusion

In the case scenario discussed at the beginning of the chapter, the hospital was found negligent because the Foley catheter had not been tested before insertion. The standard of care is to test the catheter balloon before insertion. This standard of care was introduced as evidence against the hospital [19].

Medical equipment liability poses a new challenge in an advanced technological world. There have been advancements not only in equipment but also in treatment modalities, medications, and standards. Liabilities are much greater. Knowledge, communication, and competency are key components to reducing and eliminating liabilities. Competency is the key to survival and the heart of your profession.

■ ■ ■ Pertinent Points

1. Liability is an individual's or organization's responsibility to meet the standard of care for the respective practice or profession.
2. The Safe Medical Devices Act of 1990 provides rules and regulations for safety of equipment and the reporting of serious injuries and/or deaths related to malfunctioning equipment.
3. Technological advances and complex health care continue to challenge all professions.
4. Professional codes of ethics are safeguards for professional practice.
5. Continued competency must be monitored. Incompetence must not be tolerated.
6. Competence equals professionalism.
7. Failure to communicate, failure to follow through, and failure to document are three key areas in which liability occurs.
8. Knowledge, communication, and competency are key components to reducing and/or eliminating liabilities.

■ ■ ■ Study Questions

1. Differentiate liability, strict liability, and product liability.
2. What constitutes a medical device or medical equipment?
3. What does SMDA mean?
4. Name at least three codes of ethics that are similar among the American Association of Respiratory Care, the American Physical Therapy Association, and the American Occupational Therapists Association, or your profession.
5. What should a caregiver do when he or she identifies incompetence?
6. What are common areas of medical equipment liability?
7. Identify at least five strategies for reducing and/or eliminating liabilities related to medical equipment.
8. What are common-thread "failures" to medical equipment liabilities and other liabilities?

9. Find a lawsuit in your area of practice involving equipment failure and share with your class.
10. Discuss your profession's code of ethics.
11. Share with your class policies and/or competency requirements for your area of practice.

■ ■ ■ **References**

1. Aiken, T. D. (2004). *Legal, Ethical and Political Issues in Nursing* (2nd ed.). Philadelphia: F. A. Davis Company.
2. Guido, G. W. (1997). *Legal Issues in Nursing* (2nd ed.). Stamford, Conn.: Appleton & Lange.
3. Beckmann, J. P. (1995). Problems associated with equipment and products. In *Nursing Malpractice.* Seattle: University of Washington Press.
4. Bellaire Gen. Hosp. v. Campbell, 510 S.W.2d 94 (Tex. 1974).
5. Knowlton v. Deseret Med., Inc. 930 F.2d 116, 123 (1st Cir. 1991).
6. Tammelleo, A. D. (1996). If equipment causes injury. *RN, 59*(1), 53.
7. Harris, A. V., and Ziel S. E. (1996). Reporting requirements under the Safe Medical Devices Act. *AORN Journal, 64*(3), 460.
8. Dasse, P. S. (1991, December). Commentary Improving the Safe Medical Devices Act. Online Forum. Available at http://www.rmf.org/w3961html.
9. Safe Medical Devices Act of 1990, www.fda.gov.
10. *Id.*
11. *Id.*
12. *Id.*
13. *Id.*
14. Gerlin, A. (1999, September 12). Widow's hunch reveals fatal hospital error. *The Times-Picayune Newspaper* (New Orleans), A-22.
15. Sparkman, C. (2005). Focus on healthcare delivery, quality, and nursing. *Health Policy Issues,* 82(4).
16. Smelko v. Brinton, 241 Kan. 763, 740 P.2d 591 (Kan. 1987).
17. Haddad, A. (1998). Ethics in action. *RN, 61*(9), 21.
18. Quinn, C. (1998). Infusion devices. A bleeding vein of clinical negligence. *Journal of Nursing Management, 6*(4), 209–214.
19. Pearce v. Feinstein, 754 F. Supp. 308, 309 (W.D.N.Y. 1990).

■ ■ ■ **Resources**

FDA, www.fda.gov.
Institute of Medicine, www.iom.edu.
The Joint Commission, www.jointcommission.org.
Nurse Attorney Institute, www.nurselaw.com.

12

∎∎∎

Patient Care Liability and Litigation

Key Chapter Concepts

- Allied Health Professional
- Financial Reimbursement
- Liability
- Negligence
- Nursing Home
- Patient Care
- Physical Therapy Center
- Psychiatric Center
- Rehabilitation Center

Objectives

At the conclusion of this chapter, the reader will be able to:

1. Recognize potential areas of concern or liability areas.
2. Identify negligence and a negligent act.
3. Recognize how to avoid negligence.
4. Understand the litigation process.

∎ Introduction

This chapter will explore the issues of patient care, liability, negligence, and litigation surrounding patient care.

∎ Patient Care

Patient contact is the most essential service that the allied health professional provides in the healthcare setting. The allied health professional has an obligation to practice safely and properly. At the current time, healthcare services are provided in multiple settings. Healthcare settings include the following:

1. The home, where outpatient services for an acute or chronic medical condition are provided
2. Nursing homes, long-term-care institutions that provide care for the chronically ill and elderly
3. Hospitals or medical centers, healthcare facilities where care is provided to patients who have emergency or urgent healthcare problems
4. Rehabilitation centers, short-term-care facilities where care is provided for the physically and mentally incapacitated
5. Psychiatric centers, facilities for the care of the mentally ill
6. Physical therapy centers or clinics, where outpatient recuperative services are provided

■ Documentation of Services

Financial Reimbursement

The financial reimbursement of institutions is directly associated with the services that are provided to the patients. The role of the allied health professional is to properly provide services that are ordered and to see that the services provided are documented.

Case Scenario

A patient is admitted to Columbus Hospital by his attending physician for complaints of stomach pains. The treating physician knows that the patient has a history of alcohol abuse. The physician orders that the patient be administered the medication Librium on an as-needed basis for any signs of anxiety, which is the first sign of alcohol withdrawal. If alcohol withdrawal is not controlled, the patient can become delusional and cause harm to himself or others. The attending physician has the last actual contact with the patient at 5:00 PM, at which time he leaves the patient in the hands of the nursing staff.

Although the patient initially does fairly well and is without complaint, his condition deteriorates over time. The night shift staff notice that the patient is experiencing increasing anxiety. The nursing staff does not administer Librium as ordered or call the physician to notify him of the patient's change in condition. The nurses and nurses' aides fail to closely monitor the patient.

The patient's anxiety continues. The patient clearly exhibits unusual or abnormal behavior. The patient verbally expresses anger at himself and others. He advises that he wishes to leave the hospital to buy alcohol. He refuses to comply with nursing instructions. He threatens the other patient in his room with an intravenous pole. The patient's behavior becomes so outrageous that a nurse's aide is placed outside the patient's room to keep a watchful eye on him. The patient's problem continues to escalate and ends when the patient jumps out of the window of his hospital room.

The patient falls several floors and lands on a roof extension below. Emergency services are provided. His life is saved, but he becomes a paraplegic. Before this incident, although he had an active drinking problem, he was a healthy, robust man without physical limitations or mental disability. Who is negligent? What are the negligent acts?

Documentation

Documentation of a service provided to the patient is as simple as writing a note in a patient's chart or as complex as preparing a bill for the services. Documentation of a service depends on which allied health professional provides the services. For instance, a nurse's aide or nursing assistant records vital signs. A physical, occupational, or respiratory therapist records treatment information in a patient's chart. Other allied health professionals do not document in a patient's chart but give information to a supervisor, nurse, physician's assistant, or physician, who then enters information in the patient's chart. The documentation requirements depend on the professional and on the policies and procedures of the facility.

■ Who Are Allied Health Professionals?

The **allied health professional** plays a role in providing either direct or indirect services to patients (Boxes 12-1 and 12-2). Allied health professionals who provide direct services or indirect services under the direction of a supervisor, registered nurse, dentist, physician's assistant, or physician include the following:

Box 12-1 | **Direct Services**

1. Taking vital signs
2. Performing respiratory therapy
3. Performing physical therapy
4. Performing occupational therapy

Box 12-2 | Indirect Services

1. Assisting in a medical procedure
2. Assisting a nurse in providing a treatment to a patient
3. Handing instruments to a healthcare provider who is actually performing a procedure
4. Assisting a physical therapist in the transport of a patient

1. Medical assistant
2. Respiratory therapist/respiratory technician
3. Rehabilitation/science professional, physical therapist, physical therapy assistant, occupational therapist, occupational assistant
4. Nursing assistant/nursing aide
5. Dental hygienist/dental technician
6. Imaging technologist

Examples of direct services include taking vital signs and performing respiratory therapy, physical therapy, or occupational therapy.

The allied health professional might also provide indirect services. An example of indirect services includes assisting a physician or nurse during a treatment or medical procedure.

■ Liability

Allied health professionals are liable for their negligent acts that cause injuries to patients. Liability occurs in two ways:
1. From an act or omission by an allied health professional
2. When the allied health professional participates or acts in a supervisory capacity in a negligent act committed by another healthcare provider

The allied health professional is negligent when he or she deviates from the accepted or reasonable allied health professional standard. For example, a physical therapist applies hot-pack therapy treatment to a patient's extremity. The therapist must determine whether the hot packs are of an even, consistent, and appropriate temperature to prevent patient burns. The act of applying a hot pack that burns the patient is considered negligent. The physical therapist has a duty to check the temperature before application, to ensure patient safety, and to prevent burns of extremities.

Faulty Equipment

If a nurse requests that a nursing assistant or medical assistant assist in the transport of a patient and instructs him or her to obtain a stretcher, the stretcher that is obtained should be in good working order. If the assistant knows that the stretcher has a faulty wheel but uses it anyway, the assistant may be held negligent if injury occurs. The law deems that the knowledge of faulty equipment puts the allied health professional on notice of the potential for possible injury to the patient. The nursing or medical assistant has a duty to check equipment to ensure that it is in safe working order and to report faulty equipment so that it can be repaired.

▪ ▪ ▪ What If?

You find a coworker stealing a thermal pad. He tells you that he is taking it because it does not work that well anyway and his terminally ill mother needs one.
What do you do?
What are the legal, ethical, and professional implications?

Treatment Negligence

Another example of negligence involves a respiratory therapist or technician. For example, a therapist is assigned to administer a respiratory treatment to a fresh postoperative patient, Ms. Wong, who is on the telemetry unit. However, because the therapist fails to properly identify the patient, he does not realize that there are actually two patients on the telemetry unit with the last name of Wong. The patient that the therapist administers the treatment to has an untoward reaction, which results in severe respiratory distress. The therapist is negligent for providing a treatment to the wrong patient. The therapist has a duty to properly identify a patient by checking the patient's full name, armband, or other means for patient identification. The therapist has also committed a battery by treating a patient for whom no order of treatment existed. (A battery is an intentional tort or wrongdoing. It is a harmful or offensive touching of another without his or her consent or without a legally justifiable reason.)

> **Case Discussion**
>
> An emergency room nursing assistant allegedly engaged in digital and oral sex with a patient without resistance. The patient stated while the assistant was alone in the room with her, she made sexual comments to get him to release her from restraints. She had been brought in by police for a manic-depressive disorder and was yelling, kicking, swearing, and had to be restrained. Patient told a social worker about the sexual incident three days later.
>
> Legal issue: Was the medical center liable for the actions of the nursing assistant under the theory of respondeat superior?
>
> Disposition: The jury at the trial court level awarded the plaintiff $750,000 for past damages and $500,000 for future damages. The verdict was reduced to present-day value and a judgment was rendered for $1,147,247.42. The court of appeals reversed and remanded the case for entry of a judgment of dismissal holding that the trial court erred in denying directed verdict and motion for summary judgment because the plaintiff failed to present a material question of fact regarding the defendant's liability under the legal doctrine of respondeat superior. The Supreme Court of Michigan held that court of appeals correctly reversed the trial court judgment. The plaintiff did not prove defendant was liable under the doctrine of respondeat superior. The nursing assistant was not acting within the scope of his employment when he engaged in sexual acts with the plaintiff.

Source: Zsigo v. Hurley Med. Ctr., 716 N.W.2d 220 (Mich. 2006).

Standards of Care

To determine whether the allied health professional conducted himself or herself as a reasonable professional, the judge or jury determines whether the professional practiced in accordance with the accepted standards in that particular specialty. Allied health professionals must conduct themselves in accordance with the applicable professional standards, rules, and regulations (Box 12-3).

■ Common Areas of Negligence

The allied health professional can breach the standards of care in many ways. Examples of the primary area of concern for some of the allied health professional groups are presented in Boxes 12-4 through 12-7.

Nursing and medical assistants share the same areas of potential negligence. They can avoid negligence by conducting themselves

Box 12-3 | **Sources of Standards**

The sources for standards of care include, but are not limited to, the following:
1. Allied health professional associations
2. Rules and regulations set forth by the Joint Commission
3. Policies, procedures, bylaws, rules, and regulations set forth by an institution or employer
4. Current medical literature and authoritative textbooks
5. Experts in the field
6. Job descriptions
7. Instruction manuals
8. Professional licensing boards policies/guidelines/opinions
9. State statutes and regulations
10. Equipment manuals

Box 12-4 | **Common Areas of Negligence for Nursing Assistants**

1. Failure to document, report, or record information accurately, promptly, and properly
2. Failure to properly assist a patient while ambulating, getting out of bed, or during transport
3. Failure to properly position a patient
4. Unsafe placement or positioning of equipment or medical devices
5. Failure to properly monitor a patient under observation
6. Failure to report changes in a patient's condition to a nurse or physician or other appropriate healthcare provider
7. Failure to adhere to facility rules, regulations, policies, or procedures
8. Failure to properly perform a task such as assisting a patient with feeding or bathing or providing other patient contact
9. Failure to properly provide equipment to a physician or nurse whom the aid is assisting
10. Failure to recognize equipment failure or problems resulting in patient injury

reasonably when providing patient services. The nursing or medical assistant must be careful when assisting patients and should always give adequate physical support and ensure that pathways are clear. The nursing or medical assistant who is responsible for bedridden patients must turn patients frequently and safely and comfortably position patients to avoid decubitus ulcers (bedsores). Also, documentation of these actions is key in protecting the facility and healthcare provider in a claim of medical

Box 12-5 | Common Areas of Negligence for Medical Assistants

1. Failure to properly assist a patient while ambulating, getting out of bed, or during transport
2. Failure to properly and safely position a patient
3. Unsafe placement or positioning of equipment or medical devices
4. Failure to monitor a patient during required observation
5. Failure to adhere to the employer's rules, policies, regulations, and procedures
6. Negligently providing equipment to a healthcare provider during a procedure
7. Failure to give proper advice or instructions to a patient
8. Failure to refer inquiry directly to the registered nurse, physician, or other appropriate healthcare provider

Box 12-6 | Common Areas of Negligence for Respiratory Therapists and Technicians

1. Failure to timely and properly document
2. Failure to timely and properly perform a treatment
3. Participation in a treatment that another healthcare provider performs negligently
4. Failure to properly check the working order of all equipment that is used
5. Use of faulty equipment
6. Failure to adhere to a facility's policies, procedures, practices, and protocols
7. Failure to recognize and/or report a change in respiratory status to a supervisor or physician

Box 12-7 | Common Areas of Negligence for Physical Therapists, Occupational Therapists, and Assistants

1. Failure to timely and properly document
2. Failure to timely and properly perform a treatment
3. Participation in a treatment that another healthcare provider performs negligently
4. Failure to properly check the working order of all equipment that will be used
5. Use of faulty equipment
6. Failure to adhere to a hospital's policies, procedures, practices, and protocols
7. Failure to recognize and/or report a change in status to a supervisor or the physician

negligence involving the development of a decubitus ulcer or an exacerbation of the ulcer leading to death, sepsis, amputation, or extended hospital stays. Also, when positioning a patient on an examining room table or in a bed, the assistant must protect the patient from injury.

When using equipment, the nursing and medical assistant must check the equipment to ensure that it is in good working order. The assistant is not required to act as an engineer. However, the assistant must use common sense when securing or using equipment. Equipment that has been previously known to malfunction or that has an obviously broken part should not be used. If placing equipment in a patient's room, it should be done properly and safely. Extension cords, furniture, or rugs should not be left in the patient's walkway or in areas that can cause injury or falls.

The assistant assigned to monitor the patient must do so diligently. If the patient is to be observed at set intervals, then this must be done and documented. If restraints are to be regularly checked, then the assistant needs to physically accomplish this monitoring by touching and properly observing and documenting. If a change in the patient's condition is noticed, this must also be reported to a supervisor.

Tasks should be delivered in accordance with the employer's protocols. The employer has written policies to ensure the quality of services. Policies are used to give direction to employees. For example, if assisting a patient in eating, hot beverages must not be left in unsafe positions so that they can spill on the patient.

The assistant must accurately record or provide information to a supervisor regarding a patient. If there is an obligation to document information, then it must be done in a timely fashion so that other healthcare providers have the information available to them. Assistants should not give nursing or medical instructions or advise patients. Any questions from the patient should be communicated to the nurse, physician, or other appropriate healthcare provider.

▪ ▪ ▪ **What If?**

You witness a coworker falsifying the medical record.
What do you do?
What are the legal, ethical, and professional issues?

■ Liability and Litigation

If the allied health professional acts negligently, there is a significant chance that he or she will be sued. Patients have become a litigious group. Some are quick to sue for actual wrongdoing or perceived wrongdoing. There is a high but unrealistic expectation on the part of patients that all the contact they have with the healthcare system will be positive and beneficial to them. A negative experience, even one that results in minor injury, is enough for some patients to file a lawsuit or a complaint with professional boards.

Financial compensation is a patient's redress for injuries that have been sustained. Patients can receive compensation, to name just a few, for actual physical injuries; past, present, and future medical expenses; past, present, and future lost wages; pain and suffering; emotional distress; mental anguish; and loss of consortium. If sued, you will be served with a copy of the lawsuit or a letter outlining plaintiffs, defendants, and allegations of breaches of the standard of care. Some states have a different pretrial process whereby the plaintiff must present the case to a medical review panel for review before filing the claim with the courts. The claim must be given immediately to the employer. In turn, the employer gives the paperwork to the insurance carrier. The insurance carrier then assigns an attorney to the healthcare provider. It is not unusual that the same attorney who represents the employer, the hospital, nursing home, doctor's office, or clinic also represents the allied health professional. **If you have your own professional liability policy, contact your insurance carrier immediately**.

The attorney who is assigned to you will represent your interest. Once you are sued, you should not discuss the case with anyone except your attorney. The insurance company pays all costs associated with the lawsuit, including attorneys' fees, litigation costs (e.g., for experts, documents, and exhibits), court costs, and trial costs. More important, the insurance carrier pays for any settlement of the case. It also pays a judgment if the case goes to trial and a jury awards the patient money.

To avoid being sued, the allied health professional must practice defensively. You must be vigilant and conduct yourself as a "reasonable" allied healthcare professional. If you are unsure about or do not know the policy, practices, or protocol for a specific treatment or procedure, then you must seek help from someone who is more knowledgeable.

The healthcare environment can be a dangerous environment. Many allied health professionals work in areas of health care where there is a shortage of help. Others work in critical or emergency settings, which have inherent liability because of the ever-present fast pace at which services are delivered. Everyone must respond reasonably even during times which are truly life-or-death situations. Allied health professionals may also find themselves in settings where their coworkers are not adequately trained.

▪ ▪ ▪ What If?

> While you are supervising you notice that one of the employees needs more training. If she does not receive additional training and causes injury to a patient, what are the legal and ethical consequences for her and you as the supervisor?

■ Conclusion

The allied health professional must know and identify areas of potential liability. The case scenario in this chapter indicates an area of potential liability for the nursing assistant. The nursing assistant whom nurses instructed to monitor and observe the patient failed to adequately do so. The patient jumped out of the window of his hospital room with the nurse's aide sitting immediately outside his hospital room door. The nurse's aide failed to observe a marked increase of anxiety and expression of communication by the patient of his intent to cause harm to himself. The nurse's aide failed to properly observe the patient by not watching him more closely and allowing him to exit through the hospital room window, falling and resulting in severe and permanent injury. The nurse's aide should have performed checks more frequently or should have observed the patient at his bedside. The aide should have been instructed to actually stay in the patient's room and should have promptly reported any change in the patient's condition to the supervisor.

▪ ▪ ▪ Pertinent Points

1. Being able to recognize a potential wrongdoing or negligent act and knowing the areas of potential legal exposure can decrease your involvement in litigation and potential conflicts.
2. Patient care issues and medical equipment problems are two areas of potential litigation.

3. Communication among healthcare professionals, patients, and patients' families is an important key to decreasing potential litigation.
4. Documentation is a key defense in any malpractice action.

▪ ▪ ▪ Study Questions

1. What are three areas of practice commonly breached by nursing assistants?
2. List five sources for standards of care for allied health professionals.
3. How can medical assistants decrease potential liability in their practice? Describe five ways.
4. What are things that can be done to decrease liability when using medical equipment?
5. What are five areas of potential legal exposure for the respiratory therapist technician?
6. Describe areas of negligence that you have found in a case obtained from the law library or the internet in the area of physical therapy.
7. List and describe six common healthcare settings.
8. Describe common areas of negligence where nursing assistants may be held accountable.
9. What are concerns for dental hygienists and technicians when dealing with patients?
10. Discuss how documentation can aid in defending a negligence action.
11. Find a case involving your area of practice and discuss (a) the findings and decision of the court, (b) the allegations of negligence/malpractice, and (c) what the healthcare provider could have done to decrease or prevent the chances of being involved in a lawsuit.
12. Discuss the documentation policies/procedures or national standards for your area of practices.

▪ ▪ ▪ Resources

FindLaw, www.findlaw.com.
Joint Commission, www.jointcommission.org.
Joint Commission International, www.jointcommissioninternational.com.
Legal, Ethical, and Conflict Issues for Nurses, CD-ROM interactive learning set.
Louisiana State University Health Sciences Center, www.nursing.lsuhsc.edu.
Nurse Attorney Institute, www.nurselaw.com.

13

Conflict Management and the Healthcare Provider

Key Chapter Concepts

- Alternative Dispute Resolution (ADR)
- Arbitration
- Communication
- Dispute
- Facilitation
- Facilitator
- Mediation
- Negotiation
- Nonverbal Communication
- Open-Ended Questions
- Closed-Ended Questions
- Body Language

Objectives

At the conclusion of this chapter, the reader will be able to:

1. Discuss the reasons for using alternative dispute resolution (ADR).
2. Define *negotiation*.
3. Define *mediation* and *arbitration*.
4. Define *facilitation* and *facilitative techniques*.
5. Discuss the communication process and its role in ADR.
6. Discuss common signals of body language.

■ Introduction

Disputes take the form of arguments, challenges, contests, lawsuits, fights, or even war. The **alternative dispute resolution (ADR)** movement is the process that focuses on alternative ways to resolve disputes among parties, including employers and employees or others in confrontational situations. Disputes occur constantly and are resolved daily, some in a more effective manner than others. The ability to resolve disputes at an early stage avoids the following:

1. **Lengthy court delays**
2. **Uncontrollable costs**
3. **Unwanted publicity**
4. **Ill will**
5. **Win-lose courtroom confrontation**
6. **Destruction of relationships**

In addition, quick resolution protects ongoing relationships by using impartial, neutral third parties to resolve the dispute. The ADR movement resolves conflict through the following processes:

1. **Negotiation**
2. **Mediation**
3. **Arbitration**
4. **Facilitation**
5. **Communication**

■ Negotiation

Negotiation is any communication used in an attempt to achieve a goal, approval, or action by another. Those in allied health use negotiation skills in many situations with patients, families, coworkers, and employers.

We learn the process of negotiation at a young age. When you were young and asked your parents for four cookies and they said one and you finally settled for two, you were negotiating. Negotiating takes place every time two or more individuals iron out a disagreement, an area of contention, or an area that requires some compromising on one or both sides. It may be formal or informal (Box 13-1).

■ Mediation

Mediation is the process by which a neutral third party (who may be an attorney, judge, or other person trained in mediation techniques) facilitates and assists the parties in resolving a dispute (Box 13-2). The fundamental principal of mediation is self-determination. Mediation relies on the ability of the parties to reach a voluntary, uncoerced agreement. The **mediator** may offer a

Box 13-1 | **Negotiation Skill Tips**

- Research your opponent and prepare for the negotiations.
- Determine your opponent's needs and desires.
- When negotiating, add "extras" that can be used as giveaways; you give up something and the other side can do the same.
- Know your bottom line.
- Use various techniques to negotiate effectively, such as "good cop, bad cop" role-playing.
- Watch body language—yours and your opponent's; it can reveal things not actually said.
- Confirm in writing changes that have been agreed upon by the parties.
- Negotiate in a neutral place if possible.
- Start with things that you can both agree upon to start the process.
- Have the attitude that you will "walk away" from the table if your terms are not met.

Box 13-2 | **Mediation**

The mediation process allows participants the opportunity to:
1. Address past conflicts and problems
2. Address future relationships
3. Discuss in detail problems in a nonthreatening environment
4. Make informed, voluntary, and uncoerced decisions
5. Have access to the process no matter their level of economic or societal status in the community
6. Discuss conflicts with expectations of confidentiality
7. Have access to legal counsel
8. Empower the parties to resolve disputes, as they are the decision makers

possible resolution for discussion, help parties explore options, identify issues, and provide information. There is more than one model for mediation, but most models recognize at least the following stages to the process:
1. **Introduction to the process, parties, and general rules**
2. **Information gathering**
3. **Identification of parties' interests**
4. **Brainstorming and generating of ideas and options**
5. **Negotiation and selection of appropriate resolution**
6. **Clarification and finalization of the agreement**

Both the private sector and the public sector use mediation to resolve disputes. For example, government agencies have been charged with investigating and adjudicating workplace claims. The U.S. Equal Employment Opportunity Commission, the U.S. Postal Service, and state agencies are using mediation programs as a means to end disputes. The U.S. Supreme Court has held that employment contracts may require arbitration of employer-employee disputes [1]. Mediation can also be compelled by contract.

The mediation process is commonly used to resolve medical malpractice claims, personal injury claims, and employee disputes. It is the least adversarial mode of confrontation and assists the parties in identifying the real issues and options for settlement. The parties maintain control of the outcome.

■ Arbitration

Arbitration is the process of resolving issues in conflict in a more structured setting like formal litigation. There can be one arbitrator or a panel of arbitrators that can award damages, interest, attorney's fees, and punitive damages (if allowed by law). Also, in the arbitration process, discovery is allowed and witness lists are produced. Informal rules of evidence are used. Arbitration is usually voluntary but the law can mandate it for specific disputes, such as those involving labor and unions. The arbitrator, a neutral party, should provide a written opinion and award that include the type of dispute and issues decided. Remedies should be consistent with statutes or the law that would apply if the case were tried in court.

■ Facilitation

Facilitation is the process by which a facilitator, a third party, assists in the resolution of the dispute. The types of interactive facilitative processes used to resolve contract issues include the following:

1. *Guided dialogue:* **a process used to facilitate group conversations and dialogue that allows the members of the group to share diverse perspectives in a nonconfrontational manner, and provides an environment for meaningful communication.** It is the art of asking questions that provide meaningful discussion on tough issues, broaden a group's perspective on a particular topic, and show how to elicit clear ideas and conclusions to a productive end without heated arguments.

2. *Consensus building:* **a process used to facilitate group consensus-based decisions that respects the diversity of perspective, inspire individual action, and supports an integrated view**. This facilitative process allows you to productively tap rational and intuitive thought processes, integrate diverse ideas, generate practical and innovative solutions, and facilitate individual ownership and group synergy.
3. *Action planning:* **a method of short-term planning for an event or project that has already been agreed on or about which there is already some consensus**. This is a proven implementation-planning process that enables a group to rapidly develop an effective plan, organize needed resources, and mobilize individuals' energies into action.
4. *Strategic planning:* **a process that uses facilitative strategic thinking that motivates and energizes those who will implement the plan**.
5. *Vision planning:* **a process that uses strategic thinking to develop and energize those involved to create "the big picture."**
6. *Focused conversation:* **a facilitative process that provides an environment for collective thinking to take place within a limited time frame**.
7. *The systems-change dynamics of human transformation:* **a theoretical and practical foundation of human transformation and systems change that can be used in personal and professional areas of conflict and life**. This process allows the facilitator to eliminate politics and power plays.

A trained facilitator uses the processes to guide and aid the group to reach their goals. Every participant is treated as equal and has a say in the processes used.

■ Communication

If you are in a situation in which a patient has told you that he wants to live and requests that you help him in every way possible, but he then refuses to get out of bed or take his medication, what message is he really communicating through his actions?

Communication is the process by which a person conveys his or her needs, wants, feelings, or ideas through verbal or nonverbal means. Listening is a key to effective communication. Open-ended and closed-ended questions elicit information that can be useful in the communication process and ADR (Box 13-3).

Box 13-3 | Sample Question Types

Open-Ended Questions

1. How do you feel today?
2. How are you dealing with the death of your sister?
3. How do you like the contract offered to you?
4. How can we change the way we do things to increase patient safety?
5. How are we going to decrease medication errors?

Closed-Ended Questions

1. Did you eat your breakfast?
2. Does your right foot hurt this morning?
3. Can you move your arm?
4. Where is the patient's chart?
5. Do you understand how to change your dressing?

In addition to verbal communication, the healthcare provider must be attentive to nonverbal communication. Nonverbal communication can take the form of the following:

1. **Body language with your eyes, face, hands, legs, arms, and posture**
2. **Clothing**
3. **Hygiene**

Your body language also reveals many feelings (Box 13-4): for example, rolling your eyes (as if in disbelief), tapping your fingers (anxiety), or crossing your arms (a defensive position).

Professionals also dress in a certain manner. Sloppy clothing and poor hygiene (such as uncombed hair or being unshaven) present a certain image or picture to the outside world.

▪▪▪ What if?

You are talking to a coworker about a patient's care and you notice that he will not look at you, continually tugs at his ear, and folds his arms across his chest. How do you feel? What is his body language telling you?

In ADR, the mediator or arbitrator is trained to detect body language and communication signals that can stall or cause the process to fail. It is his or her job to facilitate the process and continue to achieve progress in the negotiations and, hopefully, to conclude the matter.

Both communication and negotiation skills must be learned by the healthcare provider for use in the ADR process. ADR is a

Box 13-4 | Signals of Body Language

1. Folded arms can be a defensive action.
2. Eye contact means looking into someone's eyes to establish trust and rapport.
3. Stand and plant feet equally apart with a strong stance.
4. Avoid nervous habits, such as curling or playing with your hair, pulling on your ear or earring, and/or tapping your fingers, nail biting, kicking you leg when sitting, biting your lip, and pacing.
5. Notice the types of words used: visual, "I see what you mean"; auditory, "I hear what you're saying"; and kinesthetic, "I feel really bad for her."
6. When negotiating, sit next to each other without a desk or table between you as an obstacle so that you are equals.
7. When negotiating, "play" on the same plane; both parties should sit or stand to give the appearance of being equals.
8. Note that some people will not look at your eyes when lying.
9. If you must use a table to negotiate, use a round one so that all are equals rather than a rectangular table that has two head positions at each end.
10. When someone is speaking to you, "lean in" to show that person you are interested in what she is saying.
11. Use active listening skills.
12. Use body language that is "open" and invites the other party to talk to you.

solution to timely and efficiently conclude complicated, costly, and time-consuming conflicts in the healthcare arena.

▪ ▪ ▪ What If?

You are negotiating a new contract with a facility for a management position. You have spoken to your friend about your bottom line and what you really want.

The next day during negotiations, the facility manager seems to "know" where you are headed and your bottom line. You are furious and learn that your friend spoke to an administrator at a social event last night.
1. What are the ethical dilemmas?
2. What are the legal issues?
3. What should you do?

▪ ▪ ▪ Pertinent Points

1. Alternative dispute resolution (ADR) provides alternative ways to resolve disputes in the form of mediation, arbitration, facilitation, and negotiation.

2. Facilitation is the process by which a facilitator assists in the resolution of the dispute.
3. Healthcare providers need communication skills to effectively handle situations with patients, family, coworkers, and employer-employee conflicts.
4. Body language signals are just as important as what is actually being said.

▪▪▪ Study Questions

1. Watch a television show and identify five types of communication—verbal or nonverbal— that the characters use.
2. Develop a scenario that involves a dispute between
   a. Coworkers
   b. Employer and employee
   c. Patient and provider
   d. Insurance company and staff
      Decide and discuss how you approach resolution of the disputes.
3. Have a local facilitator or mediator talk to your class about techniques used.
4. Discuss body language and five types of signals that a person conveys through body language.
5. Have a facilitator in your area come to class and demonstrate one of the interactive facilitative processes.
6. Role-play using only nonverbal body language and discuss the interactions.
7. Find three (a) facilitation resource sites, (b) mediation resource sites, and (c) arbitration resource sites on the internet.
8. Find an internet resource on how to interpret body language.

▪▪▪ References

1. *Circuit City, Inc. v. Adams*, 532 U.S. 105 (2001).

▪▪▪ Resources

ABA, SPIDR, and AAA. Model Standards of Practice for Mediators.
Aiken, T. D. (2004). *Legal, Ethical, and Political Issues in Nursing* (2nd ed.). Philadelphia: F. A. Davis Company.
Alessandra, T. & Hunsacker, P. (1993). *Communicating at Work*. New York: Simon and Schuster.

American Arbitration Association, www.adr.org.

The American Association of Nurse Attorneys, www.taana.org.

American Bar Association, Section of Dispute Resolution, www.abanet.org.

Dauer, E. et al. (2000). *Health Care Dispute Resolution Manual: Techniques for Avoiding Litigation.* Gaithersburg, MD: Aspen Publishers.

Donaldson, M. & Donaldson, M. (1996). *Negotiating for Dummies.* Chicago: IDG Books Worldwide, Inc.

International Association of Facilitators, www.iaf-world.org.

Jean Watts Facilitative Leadership Training Institute, www.facilitativeleader.com.

Kovach, K. (1994). *Mediation Principles and Practice,* St. Paul: West Group.

Legal, Ethical, and Conflict Issues for Nurses, CD-ROM interactive learning set (published 2006). Louisiana State University Health Sciences Center School of Nursing, www.nursing.lsuhsc.edu.

Nurse Attorney Institute, www.nurselaw.com.

Society of Professionals in Dispute Resolution (SPIDR), Association for Conflict Resolution, www.acrnet.org.

Appendix A

Resource Section

American Academy of Physician Assistants
950 N. Washington St.
Alexandria, VA 22314
(703) 836-2272
Fax: (703) 684-1924
www.aapa.org

American Association of Cardiovascular and Pulmonary Rehabilitation
401 N. Michigan Ave., Suite 2200
Chicago, IL 60611
(312) 321-5146
Fax: (312) 527-6635
www.aacvpr.org

American Association of Dental Maxillofacial Radiographic Technicians
1 Scripps Dr., Suite 101
Sacramento, CA 95825
(916) 646-3740
www.aadmrt.com

American Association of Medical Assistants
20 N. Wacker Dr., Suite 1575
Chicago, IL 60606
(312) 899-1500
Fax: (312) 899-1259
www.aama-ntl.org

American Association for Respiratory Care
9425 N. MacArthur Blvd., Suite 100
Irving, TX 75063
(972) 243-2272
Fax: (972) 484-2720
www.aarc.org

American Dental Hygienists' Association

444 N. Michigan Ave., Suite 3400
Chicago, IL 60611
www.adha.org

The American Occupational Therapy Association

4720 Montgomery Lane
P.O. Box 31220
Bethesda, MD 20824
(301) 652-2682
Fax: (301) 652-7711
www.aota.org

American Physical Therapy Association

1111 N. Fairfax St.
Alexandria, VA 22314
(703) 684-2782
Fax: (703) 684-7343
www.apta.org

American Society for Clinical Pathology

1225 New York Avenue NW, Suite 250
Washington, D.C. 20005
(202) 347-4450
Fax: (202) 347-4453
(800) 267-2727
www.ascp.org

American Society of Radiologic Technologists

15000 Central Ave. SE
Albuquerque, NM 87123
(800) 444-2778
Fax: (505) 298-5063
www.asrt.org

Association of Vascular and Interventional Radiographers

12100 Sunset Hills Rd., Suite 130
Reston, VA 20190
(703) 234-4055
Fax: (703) 435-4390
www.avir.org

The Federation of State Boards of Physical Therapy
509 Wythe St.
Alexandria, VA 22314
(703) 299-3100
Fax: (703) 299-3110
www.fsbpt.org

International Society and Clinical Densitometry
342 N. Main St.
West Hartford, CT 06117
(860) 586-7563
Fax: (860) 586-7550
www.iscd.org

National Association of Emergency Medical Technicians
132-A E. Northside Dr.
Clinton, MS 39056
(601) 924-7744
(800) 34-NAEMT
Fax: (601) 924-7325
www.naemt.org

National Association of Health Care Assistants
1201 L Street NW
Washington, D.C. 20005
(800) 784-6049
www.nahcacares.org

National Board of Respiratory Care
8310 Nieman Rd.
Lenexa, KS 66214
(913) 599-4200
Fax: (913) 541-0156
www.nbrc.org

National Dental Hygienists' Association
P.O. Box 22463
Tampa, FL 33622
(800) 234-1096
www.ndhaonline.org

National Network of Career Nursing Assistants
3577 Easton Rd.
Norton, OH 44203
(330) 825-9342
Fax: (330) 825-9378
www.cna-network.org

National Rehabilitation Association
633 S. Washington St.
Alexandria, VA 22314
(703) 836-0850
Fax: (703) 836-0848
www.nationalrehab.org

Society of Diagnostic Medical Sonography
2745 Dallas Pkwy., Suite 350
Plano, TX 75093
(800) 299-9506
Fax: (214) 473-8563
www.sdms.org

Appendix B

The Trial Process

1. Prelitigation medical review panel or tribunal (does not apply in all states for medical malpractice claims)
2. Filing of the lawsuit in the appropriate state or federal court
3. Discovery: various techniques (e.g., depositions, interrogatories, requests for production of documents and things, admissions of fact, independent medical examinations) are used to discover pertinent information relating to the facts and issues of the case.
4. Pretrial settlement hearing
5. Mediation before trial
6. Trial by judge or jury
7. Appeal of the decision or judgment

Glossary

Administrative Law: Codifies interactions between citizens and government agencies, provides certain police power to the agencies to enforce the regulations, and governs the agencies themselves.

Administrative Remedies: Monetary fines, required education, loss of license to practice, or restrictions in practice.

Against Medical Advice (AMA): Refers to situations in which the patient wishes to leave the facility against physicians' advice.

Agencies: Bodies that enact rules and regulations that become administrative law.

Aggregate Amount: The total amount that the insurer pays during the policy period, usually one year, regardless of the number of incidents, claims, claimants, or defendants.

Alternative Dispute Resolution (ADR): The processes such as facilitation, mediation, and negotiation that focus on alternative ways to resolve disputes among parties, including employers and employees or others in confrontational situations.

Arbitrary: Subject to individual will or judgment without restriction; capricious.

Arbitration: The process of resolving issues in conflict in a more structured setting like formal litigation.

Assault: Placing someone in immediate fear or apprehension of a harmful or noxious touching without that person's consent; an intentional tort.

Autonomy: Independence or freedom of one's will and actions.

Battery: A harmful or offensive touching of another without his or her consent or without a legally justifiable reason; an intentional tort.

Beneficence: Doing good or kindness. In bioethical terms, the principle of beneficence means that healthcare professionals should always try to help patients and make their situation better.

Bioethics: Ethics that deal with patients and health care.

Bioethical Principles: (1) Patient's autonomy; (2) beneficence; (3) nonmaleficence; (4) justice; and (5) professional ethics.

Breach of Confidentiality: Occurs when someone who has legitimate access to health information about a patient shares it without the patient's consent with others who have no legitimate reason to know.

Checks and Balances: Limits imposed on all branches of a government by vesting in each branch the right to amend decisions of or veto another branch.

Civil Code: Developed from Roman law and codified by the legislature.

Civil Law: An individual or entity brings a case against another for harm based in tort, contract, labor, or privacy.

Claims-Made Policy: A type of professional liability insurance policy that covers injuries that occur during the policy period and when the claim is reported to the insurance company during the policy period or during the "tail" coverage.

Claims-Made Trigger: Coverage is provided for any claim made while the policy is in force.

Clinical Laboratory Improvement Amendments (CLIA): Set forth extensive conditions or standards that laboratories must meet to be certified by the U.S. Department of Health and Human Services.

Common Knowledge Exception: The defendant's negligence is so grossly apparent or the treatment is so common that a layperson can readily appraise it using his or her everyday knowledge.

Common Law: Developed on a case-by-case basis from England, when the king decided on the basis of his "divine right."

Communication: The process by which a person conveys needs, wants, feelings, or ideas through verbal or nonverbal means.

Competence: The ability to provide a level of care according to a standard of care and according to the profession's code of ethics.

Competency: The ability to understand the nature and consequences of the medical procedure.

Consent: To permit, to approve, or to comply with.

Contribution: When there are others who, although not named in a claim, bear at least some responsibility for an incident.

CPC: (1) Computerized patient record or (2) confidential personal code.

Criminal Law: The type of law whereby a state or federal government brings a case for violation of written criminal code or statute.

Declarations Page: Frequently called "dec" page in insurance jargon, where the policy lists the name(s) of the person or institution insured.

Defamation: False communication to a third party that damages a person's reputation. Libel (written) and slander (oral) communications (both quasi-intentional torts) are two forms of defamation.

Defendant: The person or entity sued.

Dental Hygienist: A licensed primary healthcare professional, oral health educator and clinician who, as a co-therapist, provides preventative, educational, and therapeutic services supporting total health for the control of oral diseases and the promotion of oral health.

Direct Services: Taking vital signs, performing respiratory therapy, engaging in physical therapy or occupational therapy.

Disciplinary Action: Action taken against a professional's license. Usually brought because the professional has endangered patient safety by causing an unsafe condition or environment for the patient.

Disciplinary Defense Insurance: Coverage provided when a health care provider is faced with disciplinary proceedings and must defend his or her license. Disciplinary Defense Insurance can provide for such things as legal fee reimbursement or payment to the attorney; wage loss reimbursement; travel, food, and lodging reimbursement; and qualified attorneys for representation. Check with your insurance company to see if Disciplinary Defense Insurance is offered as part of your policy or as a rider.

Discriminatory: Showing prejudice or partiality.

Electronic Charting: Computerized documentation.

Endorsements: Added provisions that delete or modify the coverage provided in the standard provisions or "policy jacket." The provisions, sometimes called "riders," address items that apply to the insured's specific situation.

Ethics: Declarations of what is right or wrong and of what ought to be.

Ethics Committee: Committee created to deal with ethical problems and dilemmas in the health care setting.

Excess Coverage: The amount the insurer is obligated to pay after the second policy has paid.

Exclusions: All the circumstances for which insurance coverage is not provided.

Executive Branch: President of the United States or governor of an individual state. Can propose laws, veto laws proposed by the legislature, enforce the laws, and establish agencies.

Expert: A person with knowledge, experience, and expertise in a field of practice used in litigation to support or defend litigant's position.

Expert Testimony: Generally required to establish the applicable standard of care in malpractice actions.

False Imprisonment: The unlawful detention of a person through chemical, physical, or emotional means; an intentional tort.

Felonies: More serious crimes punishable by relatively large fines and/or imprisonment for more than one year and, in some cases, death.

Flow Sheet: A table that consists of information in columns; a graphic sheet designed so that most patient data are on one form.

Focus Charting: Uses a format of having a column for the focus or problem. The note is then organized into *D* for data, *A* for action, and *R* for response.

Fourteenth Amendment: Mandates that no state shall deprive a person of life, liberty, or property without due process of law.

Good Samaritan Law: Provides immunity for those that render health care for an emergency or disaster without reimbursement.

Graphic Sheet: A document designed so that several days' worth of data are on one form (e.g., vital sign sheet listing temperature, pulse, and respirations).

Hospitals: Healthcare facilities where care is provided to patients who have emergency, urgent or long-term healthcare problems.

Incident Report: Also known as variance or occurrence report; documentation of incidents that contain an objective factual description of events. Used as a risk management tool.

Incompetence: The failing of moral commitment in upholding the code of ethics.

Indemnification: The insured contends that some other person or entity is totally responsible for an incident and, therefore, that other person or entity should reimburse or indemnify the insured for the entire amount paid to claimant(s).

Independent Contractor: A person who is self-employed and enters into contracts to provide professional services to various entities, such as hospitals, doctors' offices, and individual clients.

Indirect Services: Assisting a physician or nurse during a treatment or medical procedure.

Informed Consent: The process of providing adequate information for a patient in an understandable fashion to enable the patient to make a knowledgeable, informed decision about whether to accept or refuse a proposed treatment. Disclosure requirements include: (1) type of procedure to be performed, (2) nature and purpose of proposed treatment, (3) material risks and consequences, (4) alternatives, and (5) consequences of no treatment.

In Personam Jurisdiction: A term that means "the court has jurisdiction over the person."

In Rem Jurisdiction: A term that means "the court has jurisdiction over the property or thing itself," rather than over the people involved.

Insurance: A contract between the insured and the insurer that protects the insured from a specified loss.

Insuring Agreement of Insuring Clause: States the agreement between the insurer and the insured as to what coverage is provided. The clause briefly states what type of claim (e.g., damages due to injury) the insurer is obligated to pay and under what conditions (e.g., injury due to acts or omissions of the insured) while the policy is in force.

Intake and Output Sheets: Documentation sheets for the healthcare provider to record the intake (e.g., intravenous fluid solutions, hyperalimentation) and output (e.g., urine, feces, gastric contents).

Intentional Infliction of Emotional Distress: To establish the tort of intentional infliction of emotional distress, the plaintiff must establish that the defendant's conduct is outrageous and beyond the bounds of common decency. Insulting behavior is not enough; actions must be egregious.

Intentional Torts: Require that there be an intentional interference with one's person, reputation, or property (e.g., assault, battery, false imprisonment).

Interrogatories: Written questions that must be answered under oath.

Invasion of Privacy: The tort of unjustifiably intruding on another's right of privacy by appropriating his or her name or likeness, unreasonably interfering with his or her seclusion, publishing private facts, or publicly placing a person in a false light; a quasi-intentional tort.

JCAHO: Joint Commission on Accreditation of Healthcare Organizations.

Judicial Branch: Court system; interprets legislation and may overrule laws and actions of the executive branch.

Judicial System: The court system (including federal courts and state courts) that develops and interprets statutory law.

Justice: Treating everyone fairly.

Kardex: An abbreviated listing of the care elements specific to the patient. The Kardex commonly defines the type of diet, the patient's activity level, the amount of assistance the patient needs for bathing, and the treatments to be performed.

Law: The foundation of statutes, rules, and regulations that govern people, relationships, behaviors, and interactions with the state, society, and federal government.

Legislative Branch: The U.S. House of Representatives and Senate and any similar state legislature that develops statutory law.

Liability: An individual's responsibility of his or her conduct for failure to meet a standard of care or for failure to perform a duty that causes harm to a client.

Liability Insurance: Insurance that protects personal and professional assets in the event of professional liability and malpractice suit.

Libel: Written defamatory statements.

Living Will: A document, which may be handwritten, in which the patient describes his or her wishes regarding life-sustaining treatment. The document only takes effect if (1) it complies with the requirements of the law of the state in which the patient is located and (2) the patient is no longer able to make healthcare decisions.

Malpractice: Dereliction of professional duty through negligence, ignorance, or criminal intent.

Mediation: The process in which a neutral third party (e.g., healthcare provider, attorney, judge, or other person trained in mediation techniques) facilitates and assists parties in resolving a dispute.

Medical Device: A broad term encompassing such items as implants, single-use disposable devices, instruments, machines, apparatus, and reagents.

Minor: An individual younger than 18.

Misdemeanors: Lesser crimes with usually modest fines or penalties established by the state or federal government and/or imprisonment of less than 1 year.

Moral Dilemma: Occurs when moral ideas conflict.

Morals: Ideas about right and wrong.

Negligence: The failure to use such care as a reasonably prudent and careful person would use under similar circumstances; an act of omission or commission or failure to do what a person of ordinary prudence would have done under similar circumstances.

Elements of Negligence: (1) Duty, (2) breach of duty, (3) proximate cause or causal connection, and (4) harm or damage.

Negotiation: Any communication used in an attempt to achieve a goal, approval, or action by another.

Nonmaleficence: Do no harm; in bioethical terms, the principle of nonmaleficence means that healthcare professionals should avoid harming a patient.

Nursing Home: A long-term-care institution that provides care for the chronically ill and elderly.

Occurrence Policy: Professional liability insurance policy that covers injuries that occur during the period covered by the policy even though they may be reported outside the policy period.

Ordinary Negligence: Conduct that involves undue risk of harm to others.

OSHA: Occupational Safety and Health Administration.

Physical Therapy Centers: Where outpatient recuperative and rehabilitative services are provided.

PIE Charting: Structures the progress note into *P* for problem, *I* for intervention, and *E* for evaluation.

Plaintiff: The person or entity bringing the suit or claim.

Plan of Care: May be recorded in a hospital or nursing home in the form of a nursing care plan; usually defines the patient's problems, the outcomes or goals to be achieved, and interventions or steps to be carried out to achieve the outcomes.

Policy Provisions: Sometimes called the "policy jacket," sets forth the generic provisions found in most policies of the same type.

Precedent: A legal decision serving as an authoritative rule in similar cases that follow.

Premium: Money that each insured member contributes that is pooled by the insurer.

Prior Acts: Incidents that occurred before the beginning effective date of the policy.

Private Institutions: Are not supported by state revenues and typically receive financial support from private funding.

Product Liability: Different from malpractice in that the patient may not have to prove a deviation from a standard of care if the courts apply a strict liability standard. With a strict liability standard, the manufacturer of the equipment, drug, or medical device may be held liable.

Professional Negligence: A negligent act or omission by a healthcare provider in the rendering of professional services that is the proximate cause of a personal injury or wrongful death, provided that the services are within the scope of services for which the provider is licensed and that are not within any restriction imposed by the licensing agency or licensed hospital.

Psychiatric Centers: Facilities for the treatment of psychiatric disorders and illness.

Public Academic Institutions: Are affiliated with state government, are deemed state institutions, and are supported by state revenues.

Radiology Technologists: Usually employed in hospitals and cancer centers to deliver radiation to patients for therapeutic purposes.

Rehabilitation Centers: Short-term-care facilities where care is provided for the physically and mentally incapacitated.

Res Ipsa Loquitur: Legal doctrine that means "the thing speaks for itself"; often used in operating room malpractice cases where sponges, needles, or hemostats are left in the patient.

Respondeat Superior: Legal doctrine that means "let the master answer"; used to hold the employer responsible and liable for the negligent acts of its employees.

Safe Medical Device Act of 1990 (SMDA): Provides rules and regulations for the safety and reporting of medical devices.

Self-insurance: Insurance of healthcare institutions that set aside sufficient funds to satisfy a successful claim instead of obtaining a policy through an insurance company for a specified amount.

Slander: Spoken defamatory statements. A quasi-intentional tort based on speech.

SOAP Format: This system consists of a problem list and progress notes. The problem list is an ongoing listing of the patient's current and resolved problems. The progress note is broken down into four components: *S* (subjective), *O* (objective), *A* (assessment), and *P* (plan).

Sovereign Immunity: A defense that protects a federal or state employee when acting within the scope of employment.

Spoliation: The intentional destruction of evidence that, when established, allows the court to instruct the jury that it may infer that the lost or damaged evidence was unfavorable to the party responsible for the spoilation.

Standard of Care: A measure of the care that a reasonable and sensible person would use in the same situation.

Stare Decisis: "To stand by things decided" or to adhere to a decided case.

Statement of the Agreement: Often called "insuring agreement" or "insuring clause"; states the agreement between the insurer and the insured as to the coverage provided.

Statute of Limitations: Used as a defense to a tort action; requires that a claim be filed within a specific amount of time.

Statutory Law: Laws that are codified and affect all citizens of the state.

Subpoena Duces Tecum: A document that attorneys direct to a custodian commanding the custodian to appear for a deposition and produce a patient's treatment record or other pertinent documents. State and federal courts have specific rules addressing the proper form, appropriate service, and other requirements necessary for the subpoena to be valid.

Surrogate Decision Maker: A person permitted under state law to consent to medical treatment on a patient's behalf when the patient is incapable of doing so.

Tail Coverage Policy: An uninterrupted extension of the insurance policy period, also known as the extended reporting endorsement.

Tort: A civil wrong, other than breach of contract; a tort is a harm against a person, whereas a crime is a harm against the state.

Trespass to Land: Occurs when a person, without the consent of the landowner, enters onto another's land or causes anyone or anything to enter the land or premises.

Umbrella Coverage: Insurance purchased in addition to basic liability policy; provides additional limit amounts and/or adds coverage for events not covered in the basic policy.

Vicarious Liability: Wherein the acts or omissions of the employee are imputed to the employer, so that the employer can be found liable for them.

X-Ray Technician or Radiographer: Uses ionizing radiation for diagnostic purposes and has specific training to perform X-rays of the chest, extremities, gastrointestinal (GI), genitourinary (GU), leg-podiatric, skull, or torso-skeletal categories.

Index